Quick &
Delicious
Diabetic
Desserts

Mary Jane Finsand

Foreword by
James D. Healy, M.D., F.A.A.P.

 Sterling Publishing Co., Inc.   New York

Edited by Laurel Ornitz

Recipe consultant: Carol Tiffany

Library of Congress Cataloging-in-Publication Data

Finsand, Mary Jane.
    Quick & delicious diabetic desserts / Mary Jane Finsand.
       p.   cm.
    Includes index.
    ISBN 0-8069-8304-3
      1. Diabetes—Diet therapy—Recipes.   2. Desserts.   I. Title.
    II. Title: Quick and delicious diabetic desserts.
    RC662.F568   1992
641.8'6—dc20   91-44523
                                                     CIP

10 9 8 7 6 5 4 3

Published in 1992 by Sterling Publishing Company, Inc.
387 Park Avenue South, New York, N.Y. 10016
© 1992 by Mary Jane Finsand
Distributed in Canada by Sterling Publishing
% Canadian Manda Group, P.O. Box 920, Station U
Toronto, Ontario, Canada M8Z 5P9
Distributed in Great Britain and Europe by Cassell PLC
Villiers House, 41/47 Strand, London WC2N 5JE, England
Distributed in Australia by Capricorn Link Ltd.
P.O. Box 665, Lane Cove, NSW 2066
Manufactured in the United States of America
All rights reserved

Sterling ISBN 0-8069-8304-3

Contents

Foreword

Quick & Delicious Diabetic Desserts is written specifically for the diabetic, but it is an excellent reference for all health-conscious people interested in adding speed and variety to their meals.

Mary Jane Finsand's other diabetic cookbooks are used and recommended by a large number of doctors, hospitals, clinics, diabetics, and diabetic organizations because the recipes are medically sound and easy to prepare. For this book, Mary Jane has developed many new and exciting ways of using common products that require little preparation. This cookbook will help diabetics add more variety to their meals, while still following their doctor's recommendations, balancing food nutrients, and adhering to a reduced-sugar diet.

Each recipe includes calories, carbohydrates, and exchanges, allowing diabetics and others to regulate their food intake according to their doctor's recommendations. Please share this cookbook with your own doctor, pharmacy, hospital dietitian, and diabetic organization. I am confident that they will confirm my high recommendation.

James D. Healy, M.D., F.A.A.P.

A Note from Covenant Medical Center

This cookbook is the resource our patients have been waiting for. As diabetes educators, we realize that adherence to the treatment regimen is increased if it can be made easier and more enjoyable, and this book does both.

Diabetics are reminded that these dessert items still need to be substituted into the diabetes meal plan. Fructose or other sugar replacements will raise blood glucose, but because less of it is needed to make an acceptable product, a smaller increase in blood glucose occurs, as compared to the effects of sucrose in a similar product. Nevertheless, we encourage diabetics to perform self–blood-glucose-monitoring to discover what effects these new items have on their blood-glucose control.

At the Diabetes Health Center at Covenant Medical Center, we recommend cookbooks that include nutritional analysis, diabetes exchanges, and tested recipes, and that have a credible author. We have found this book, as well as other cookbooks by Mary Jane Finsand, to meet that criteria.

For more information on the diabetes diet, contact a registered dietitian at your local hospital.

Mary Steffensmeier, R.D.
Lynette Gersema, R.N.
Covenant Medical Center
Waterloo, Iowa

Introduction

Most of us are always looking for ways to add more hours to the day and make the hours that we do have more productive. With so many of us working full time, five or six days a week, our time is definitely limited. It isn't easy to concoct a dessert within a limited time frame. But rather than skipping desserts altogether, we need to know what products we can use to make quick desserts to enhance our meals.

In this book, the desserts are generally easy and quick to make. The recipes have been developed using mixes or other quick common ingredients. Many of the desserts you can complete well in advance, like cookies, or cakes that you can cut into individual-serving slices, and then freeze. Some can be partially prepared beforehand and then, with a few last-minute garnishes, finished at serving time. Others are as simple as taking the ingredients from your refrigerator and assembling them.

I dedicate this book to all the busy people who want to feel their very best by following their individual diets, whether diabetic or otherwise. I hope these quick and delicious recipes will bring joy and good eating to you and your family.

Mary Jane Finsand

Sugar & Sugar Replacements

If you are a diabetic, your diet has probably been prescribed by a doctor or diet counsellor who has determined your diet requirements by considering your exercise and other daily life patterns. Do not try to outguess your doctor or counsellor. Always stay within the guidelines of your individual diet, and be sure to ask about any additions or substitutions. If you have any questions about any diabetic recipes or exchanges, ask your diet counsellor.

A recent report stated that diabetics could eat table sugar (sucrose) made from cane or beets. The research found that refined sugar did not get into the blood any more quickly than sugar from wheat flour or potatoes, and contended that because these products are starches, they could all be eaten at mealtime. However, the report also stated that the number of calories consumed must be held constant to the prescribed diet. This is one of the primary reasons why diabetics have been advised to avoid products containing refined table sugar.

Sugar has approximately 770 calories per cup with 199 grams of carbohydrates, whereas refined wheat flour has approximately 420 calories per cup with 88 grams of carbohydrates and the rest of the calories made up from the 12 grams of protein. Therefore, you would have to eat 2.26 times the amount of wheat flour to gain the same amount of grams of carbohydrates you would gain from one cup of sugar. But if you use one of the sugar replacements or new natural sweeteners on the market, you cut out most of the carbohydrates and calories normally gained when using a cane or beet sugar.

Another factor that the diabetic must consider is that later studies in the same report showed that consumption of refined table sugar results in a roller-coaster effect on the blood-glucose levels. Further studies examined the effects of fructose, a fruit sugar, on the blood-glucose levels. These studies found that fructose does not set up a mechanism that results in rapid upward surges of the blood-glucose levels. They also found the sweetening intensity of fructose to be greater than that of refined table sugar. Thus, it was concluded that fructose was a safe product for diabetics. The recipes in this cookbook are sweetened with fructose and other sugar replacements.

Most sugar replacements can be found in your supermarket. They vary in sweetness, aftertaste, aroma, and calories. The listing that follows is by ingredient name rather than product name. When you are shopping, check the side of the box or bottle to determine the contents of the product.

Aspartame and aspartame products are fairly new additions to the supermarket. Aspartame is a natural protein sweetener. Because of its intense sweetness, it reduces calories and carbohydrates in the diet. Aspartame has a sweet aroma and no aftertaste. It seems to complement some of the other sweeteners by removing their bitter aftertaste. Aspartame does lose some of its sweetness in heating, and is therefore recommended for use in cold products.

Cyclamates and products containing cyclamates are not as sweet as saccharin and saccharin products, and also leave a bitter aftertaste. Many sugar replacements consist of a combination of saccharin and cyclamates.

Fructose is commonly known as fruit sugar. It is actually a natural sugar found in fruits and honey. Fructose tastes the same as common table sugar (sucrose), but because of its intense sweetness, it reduces calories and carbohydrates in the diet. It is not affected by heating or cooling, but baked products made with fructose tend to be heavier.

Glycyrrhizen and products containing glycyrrhizen are as sweet as saccharin and saccharin products. They are seen less in supermarkets because they tend to give food a licorice taste and aroma.

Saccharin and products containing saccharin are the most widely known and used intense sweeteners. When used in baking or cooking, saccharin has a lingering bitter aftertaste. You will normally find it in the form of sodium saccharin in products labelled low-calorie sugar replacements. Granular, or dry, sugar replacements containing sodium saccharin give less of an aftertaste to foods that are heated. But it's best to use liquid sugar replacements containing sodium saccharin in cold foods or in foods that have partially cooled and no longer need any heating.

Sorbitol is used in many commercial food products. It has little or no aftertaste and a sweet aroma. At present it can only be bought in bulk form at health-food outlets.

Stevia Rebaudian is a new herb sweetener that is hundreds of times sweeter than common table sugar. It is stable when heated and retains its sweetening properties.

If you have difficulty finding these products, you can try contacting a distributor or mail-order outlet.

For the individual consumer, write:

The Fruitful Yield
2111 N. Bloomingdale Road
Glendale Hts, IL 60139

or

T & K Health Foods
1429 West 3rd St.
Waterloo, IA 50701

For health-food retailers or other large orders, write or call:

NOW Natural Foods
2000 Bloomingdale Road, Unit 250
Glendale Hts, IL 60139
Phone: (708) 893-1330

Using the Recipes— Conversion Guides, Flavorings & Extracts, Spices & Herbs

All the recipes have been developed using granulated or liquid sugar replacements. Read the recipes carefully; then assemble all equipment and ingredients. Use standard measuring equipment (whether metric or customary), and be sure to measure accurately.

Customary Terms

t.	teaspoon	qt.	quart
T.	tablespoon	oz.	ounce
c.	cup	lb.	pound
pkg.	package	°F	degrees Fahrenheit
pt.	pint	in.	inch

Metric Symbols

mL	millilitre	°C	degrees Celsius
L	litre	mm	millimetre
g	gram	cm	centimetre
kg	kilogram		

Conversion Guide for Cooking Pans and Casseroles

Customary	Metric
1 qt.	1 L
2 qt.	2 L
3 qt.	3 L

Oven-Cooking Guides

Fahrenheit °F	Oven Heat	Celsius °C
250–275°	very slow	120–135°
300–325°	slow	150–165°
350–375°	moderate	175–190°
400–425°	hot	200–220°
450–475°	very hot	230–245°
475–500°	hottest	250–290°

Use this candy-thermometer guide to test for doneness:

Fahrenheit °F	Test		Celsius °C
230–234°	Syrup:	Thread	100–112°
234–240°	Fondant/Fudge:	Soft ball	112–115°
244–248°	Caramels:	Firm ball	118–120°
250–266°	Marshmallows:	Hard ball	121–130°
270–290°	Taffy:	Soft crack	132–143°
300–310°	Brittle:	Hard crack	149–154°

Guide to Approximate Equivalents

Customary				Metric	
Ounces Pounds	Cups	Tablespoons	Teaspoons	Millilitres	Grams Kilograms
			¼ t.	1 mL	1g
			½ t.	2 mL	
			1 t.	5 mL	
			2 t.	10 mL	
½ oz.		1 T.	3 t.	15 mL	15 g
1 oz.		2 T.	6 t.	30 mL	30 g
2 oz.	¼ c.	4 T.	12 t.	60 mL	
4 oz.	½ c.	8 T.	24 t.	125 mL	
8 oz.	1 c.	16 T.	48 t.	250 mL	
2.2 lb.					1 kg

Keep in mind that this guide does not show exact conversions, but it can be used in a general way for food measurement.

Guide to Baking-Pan Sizes

Customary	Metric	Holds	Holds (Metric)
8-in pie.	20-cm pie	2 c.	600 mL
9-in. pie	23-cm pie	1 qt.	1 L
10-in. pie	25-cm pie	1¼ qt.	1.3 L
8-in. round	20-cm round	1 qt.	1 L
9-in. round	23-cm round	1½ qt.	1.5 L
8-in. square	20-cm square	2 qt.	2 L
9-in. square	23-cm square	2½ qt.	2.5 L
9 × 5 × 2 in. loaf	23 × 13 × 5 cm loaf	2 qt.	2 L
9-in. tube	23-cm tube	3 qt.	3 L
10-in. tube	25-cm tube	3 qt.	3 L
10-in. Bundt	25-cm Bundt	3 qt.	3 L
9 × 5 in.	23 × 13 cm	1½ qt.	1.5 L
10 × 6 in.	25 × 16 cm	3½ qt.	3.5 L
11 × 7 in.	27 × 17 cm	3½ qt.	3.5 L
13 × 9 × 2 in.	33 × 23 × 5 cm	3½ qt.	3.5 L
14 × 10 in.	36 × 25 cm	cookie tin	
15½ × 10½ × 1 in.	39 × 25 × 3 cm	jelly roll	

Flavorings and Extracts

Orange, lime, and lemon peels give pastries and puddings a fresh clean flavor. Liquor flavors, such as brandy and rum, give cakes and other desserts a company flair. Choose from the following to give your recipes some zip, without adding calories.

Almond	Butter rum	Pecan
Anise (Licorice)	Cherry	Peppermint
Apricot	Chocolate	Pineapple
Banana creme	Coconut	Raspberry
Blackberry	Grape	Rum
Black walnut	Hazelnut	Sassafras
Blueberry	Lemon	Sherry
Brandy	Lime	Strawberry
Butter	Mint	Vanilla
Butternut	Orange	Walnut

Spices and Herbs

These are some of my favorite spices and herbs. They will definitely add distinction to your desserts, without adding calories.

Allspice: cinnamon, ginger, and nutmeg flavor; used in breads, pastries, jellies, jams, and pickles.

Anise: licorice flavor; used in candies, breads, fruit, wine, and liqueurs.

Cinnamon: pungent, sweet flavor; used in pastries, breads, pickles, wine, beer, and liqueurs.

Clove: pungent, sweet flavor; used in ham, sauces, pastries, puddings, fruit, wine, and liqueurs.

Coriander: bitter-lemon flavor; used in cookies, cakes, pies, puddings, fruit, and wine and liqueur punches.

Ginger: strong, pungent flavor; used in anything sweet, also with beer, brandy, and liqueurs.

Nutmeg: sweet, nutty flavor; used in pastries, puddings, and vegetables.

Woodruff: sweet, vanilla flavor; used in wines and punches.

Tips & Tricks from My Kitchen

I receive many questions on cookware, bakeware, and small appliances. In this section I will give you some idea of what I have found to work best for me. Also, I will discuss alternative methods and appliances to use when you don't have a particular appliance called for in a recipe, such as a food processor or blender.

First of all, I cannot fully express the importance of using heavy bakeware. Heavy bakeware absorbs, retains, and distributes heat evenly. Many of the lighter-weight cake pans and cookie sheets have dead or hot spots in them. I have found that, in cooking with fructose, a heavy, very shiny aluminum surface produced the best, most uniform desserts.

While I do use the newer dark bakeware, I rarely consider that any bakeware with a synthetic self-releasing or nonstick surface truly has a nonstick surface. Also, I find that the dark bakeware requires different baking temperatures and times. (Remember, dark colors absorb heat.) So, if you do use dark bakeware, you might want to lower the temperature and watch your item very closely near the end of its baking time. Because I have a tendency to scratch the bottom and sides of pans, nonstick pans don't last as long for me. In addition, I found that products baked in the darker bakeware were smaller, heavier, and crispier than I wanted.

It is important that baking sheets and pans be kept clean and free from burns. Burned surfaces on baking sheets or pans prevent heat from distributing evenly, causing baked products to brown improperly. Items baked on burned sheets can come out of the oven underdone, overdone, or burned.

When baking a cake, use a heavy aluminum pan. Line the bottom with wax paper. Do not grease or flour the sides. Fill and bake as directed. After cooling slightly, release the sides by running a flexible spatula between the edges of the pan and the cake. Try to keep the edge of the spatula pressed tightly against the sides of the pan. Place a rack over the cake pan and

14

invert. Remove the wax paper, place another rack over the cake, and invert. Cool completely.

I have found that the easiest method of cutting a cake into layers is to mark the layer by sticking toothpicks around the cake at the level you want the layer. Then use a long sharp knife or a piece of thread to cut through the cake at that level. If you are cutting into three layers, mark and cut each layer separately.

Many cookware sets do not come with a double boiler. A double boiler consists of two pans, with the top pan sitting on the bottom pan. A simple double boiler can be made by placing a heat-proof bowl over a saucepan. The water in the bottom of the double boiler should not boil, just simmer.

I found that when I was cooking the instant puddings, a wire whisk produced the best results.

If you don't have a food processor or blender and want to chop an ingredient such as nuts, use a heavy knife. If you want to crush crackers or dry bread into crumbs, place broken pieces into a plastic bag and crush with your hand or a rolling pin.

You don't need a crepe iron to make crepes; a 6-in. frying pan will work. Heat a pan lightly sprayed with vegetable oil. Then remove the pan and place about 1 T. (15 mL) of batter in the pan, curl the pan until the batter coats the bottom, return to the heat, and fry lightly.

Fresh-Fruit Desserts

The beauty of fresh-fruit desserts is that they are easy, nutritious, and filling due to their high-fibre content. Selecting fresh fruit for plain eating and making desserts is the same. Although many of us are blessed with fresh fruit in the produce department of our supermarket every season of the year, every fruit has its own season, and that is when the fruit is at its succulent best. Normally, purchase your fresh fruit just before the time you are going to use it. If you are buying unripe fruit, ask how long it will take to ripen so that you can plan its use. When selecting fruit, look at its color and look for bruises, check or feel for firmness, and smell the fruit for a fresh delicate sweet aroma.

Nectarine with Pistachio Cream

1 T.	pistachio-flavored sugar-free instant pudding mix	15 mL
⅔ c.	skim milk	180 mL
2	nectarines	2
4 t.	nonfat strawberry yogurt	20 mL

Combine pistachio pudding mix and milk in a small mixing bowl. Beat with a fork or whipping whisk for 1 to 2 minutes or until well blended. Set aside for 5 to 8 minutes to allow to thicken. (Mixture should be a light-syrup consistency.) Divide and spread pistachio mixture on the bottom of four small dessert plates. Cut nectarines in half. Cut each half into ten very thin slices. Arrange slices in a fan fashion on one side of the plate on top of the pistachio mixture. Place a 1-t. (5-mL) "dot" of strawberry yogurt at the base of the nectarine fan. Chill or serve immediately.

Yield: 4 servings
Exchange, 1 serving: ½ fruit, ¼ skim milk
Calories, 1 serving: 50
Carbohydrates, 1 serving: 12 g

Nectarine with Rum Creme

1	nectarine	1
½ c.	nonfat plain yogurt	125 mL
1 env.	aspartame low-calorie sweetener	1 env.
¼ t.	rum extract	2 mL

Divide nectarine in half and remove seed. Slice each half into eight slices and arrange each half on a plate in a daisy petal–type design. Combine yogurt, sweetener, and rum extract in a small bowl. Stir to completely blend. Divide mixture evenly between the two plates, spooning it into the middle of the two daisy forms.

Yield: 2 servings
Exchange, 1 serving: ½ fruit, ¼ skim milk
Calories, 1 serving: 52
Carbohydrates, 1 serving: 11 g

Nectarine with Strawberry Sauce

1	nectarine, cubed	1
4 t.	all-natural strawberry preserves	20 mL
1 T.	prepared nondairy whipped topping	15 mL

Divide the nectarine cubes evenly and place them in two dishes. Spoon strawberry preserves into a small microwave or heat-proof dish. Heat until melted. Pour warmed preserves over nectarine cubes. Top with nondairy whipped topping. Serve immediately.

Yield: 2 servings
Exchange, 1 serving: ¾ fruit
Calories, 1 serving: 45
Carbohydrates, 1 serving: 11 g

Perfect Dates

10	soft dates	10

Pour boiling water over the dates. Allow to plump for 10 minutes. Drain and dry dates thoroughly. Place each date in a decorative petit-four case. Arrange on a small dessert plate.

Yield: 10 servings
Exchange, 1 serving: ⅓ fruit
Calories, 1 serving: 22
Carbohydrates, 1 serving: 6 g

Apple Plum Cups

1	Granny Smith apple, peeled	1
3	plums	3
1 jar	Dutch Apple Dessert strained baby food	1 jar
(4-oz.)		(113-g)
6	strawberries	6

Core apple and slice into bite-size chunks. Cut plums in half, remove seed, and cut into bite-size chunks. Combine apple and plum chunks in a glass bowl. Add Dutch Apple Dessert and toss gently to mix. Divide mixture between six cups or cup-type glasses. Slice each strawberry from the tip to the base, and spread into a fan. Place across top of mixture in cup.

Yield: 6 servings
Exchange, 1 serving: ½ fruit
Calories, 1 serving: 30
Carbohydrates, 1 serving: 8 g

Hawaiian Delight

1	pineapple	1
1	papaya	1
1	orange	1
2	bananas	2
¼ c.	chopped macadamia nuts	60 mL

Cut pineapple in half lengthwise through the crown. Use a sharp thin knife to cut the fruit out of the half shells. Wrap shells in plastic wrap; refrigerate. Remove core from pineapple fruit and cut fruit into bite-size pieces; then place in a bowl. Peel and halve papaya. Remove seeds and cut fruit into bite-size pieces. Add to pineapple in bowl. Remove peel and white membrane from orange, holding orange over the fruit bowl to catch the orange juice. Cut orange segments free and place in bowl. Mix gently. Cover bowl with plastic wrap. To serve: Slice bananas into the fruit bowl. Mix gently. Pile fruit into the two pineapple shells. Sprinkle each filled shell evenly with macadamia nuts. Serve immediately.

Yield: 10 servings (5 from each shell)
Exchange, 1 serving: 1 fruit, ½ fat
Calories, 1 serving: 71
Carbohydrates, 1 serving: 14 g

Kiwi and Pineapple with Raspberry Dip

1	kiwi, peeled and sliced	1
1	pineapple ring	1
2 T.	low-fat raspberry yogurt	30 mL

Arrange kiwi slices on one side edge of a dessert plate. Place pineapple ring slightly over the inside edge of the kiwi slices. (Pineapple ring should be approximately in middle of plate.) Spoon raspberry yogurt into the hole of the pineapple ring. Cover and chill or serve immediately.

Yield: 2 servings
Exchange, 1 serving: 1 fruit
Calories, 1 serving: 56
Carbohydrates, 1 serving: 12 g

Blueberry Glaze on Melon

¼	cantaloupe, peeled	¼
½ c.	fresh blueberries, washed	125 mL
2 T.	all-natural blueberry preserves	30 mL

Cut cantaloupe into four slices; then arrange in a double circle on a serving plate. Place blueberries in the middle of the circle. Melt blueberry preserves in a small bowl in the microwave or small saucepan. Pour liquid preserves lightly over the melon and blueberries.

Yield: 1 serving
Exchange, 1 serving: 2 fruit
Calories, 1 serving: 128
Carbohydrates, 1 serving: 28 g

Berry Bliss

1 qt.	strawberries	1 L
1 pt.	raspberries	500 mL
8 oz.	low-fat plain yogurt	240 g

Clean strawberries and arrange in a pyramid on a serving dish. Clean raspberries and whirl in a blender or food processor until a puree is formed. Add yogurt. Slightly blend. Pour over strawberry pyramid.

Yield: 6 servings
Exchange, 1 serving: 1 fruit, ¼ fat
Calories, 1 serving: 84
Carbohydrates, 1 serving: 16 g

Chocolate Apple Slices

½ c.	semisweet chocolate chips	125 mL
½ t.	brandy flavoring	2 mL
2	red apples, cored, cut into 24 wedges	2
2 T.	lemon juice	30 mL

Line a large cookie sheet with wax paper. Melt chocolate in a small heavy pan over very low heat, stirring until smooth. Mix in brandy flavoring. Remove from heat. Place apple wedges in a bowl. Sprinkle with lemon juice and toss gently. Drain and dry apple wedges thoroughly. Place a toothpick in each apple wedge. Dip one slice at a time into the melted chocolate, tipping pan as necessary. Shake excess chocolate back into pan. Place on wax paper–lined cookie sheet. Refrigerate until chocolate sets, about 1 hour.

Yield: 24 slices or servings
Exchange, 1 serving: ⅓ fruit, ⅕ fat
Calories, 1 serving: 28
Carbohydrates, 1 serving: 3 g

Berries with Lemon Custard

3 c.	strawberries, hulled and quartered lengthwise	750 mL
2 env.	aspartame low-calorie sweetener	2 env.
1 t.	grated lemon peel	5 mL
1 recipe	"Lemon Custard" (page 22)	1 recipe

Mix strawberries, aspartame sweetener, and lemon peel in a bowl. Refrigerate 3 to 4 hours or overnight. Spoon ¼ c. (60 mL) of the "Lemon Custard" into the middle of a dessert plate. Drain berries and spoon over custard. Top with remaining custard.

Yield: 6 servings
Exchange, 1 serving: ⅔ low-fat milk, ⅓ fruit
Calories, 1 serving: 87
Carbohydrates, 1 serving: 7 g

White Chocolate–Dipped Strawberries

| ½ c. | dietetic white chocolate chips | 125 mL |
| 24 | large strawberries with stems | 24 |

Line a cookie sheet with wax paper. Melt white chocolate in double boiler over very low heat, stirring until smooth. Remove from heat. Holding one strawberry at a time from the stem, dip halfway into chocolate, tipping pan if necessary. Shake excess chocolate back into pan. Place on prepared cookie sheet. Refrigerate until chocolate sets, about 30 minutes.

Yield: 24 strawberries or 8 servings
Exchange, 1 serving: ⅓ fruit, ⅕ fat
Calories, 1 serving: 25
Carbohydrates, 1 serving: 3 g

Double Chocolate with Raspberries

For Dark Chocolate Sauce:

¼ c.	semisweet chocolate chips	60 mL
3 T. + 1 t.	low-fat milk	50 mL

Fill a small saucepan with about ¾ in. of water. Bring water to a simmer. Place chocolate chips in a custard cup. Place custard cup in the simmering water. When the chips just begin to melt, add 1 T. (15 mL) of the milk. Cook and stir until mixture is smooth and creamy. Continue stirring and slowly add remaining milk. Remove custard cup from water and set aside.

For White Chocolate Sauce:

¼ c.	white chocolate chips	60 mL
3 T. + 1 t.	low-fat milk	50 mL

Proceed as for "Dark Chocolate Sauce."

Berries:

90	fresh raspberries	90

To serve:

Measure 2 t. (10 mL) of each chocolate sauce onto a small dessert plate or saucer, with dark chocolate on one side of plate and white chocolate on the other. Gently pull the tips of a fork through both sauces to give a spiral appearance. Decorate each plate of the swirled chocolate sauces with 15 raspberries. Serve immediately.

Yield: 6 servings
Exchange, 1 serving: ⅓ fruit, 1 fat
Calories, 1 serving: 92
Carbohydrates, 1 serving: 5 g

Puddings & Custards

With their smooth creamy texture and subtle flavors, puddings and custards are always a welcome conclusion to any meal. They are truly a cook's dream dessert. They can be ready almost immediately. Creamy puddings are easy to prepare, and with the addition of flavorings, they have endless possibilities. To make the best possible pudding, be sure your refrigerated set pudding is completely cooled before you cover it.

There are only two drawbacks that I have found with pudding mixes. Do not make them too far ahead of serving time; by this I mean, several days. And they do not freeze well; both the smooth texture and the delicate taste suffer from freezing.

Lemon Custard

1 pkg. (4-serving)	vanilla-flavored sugar-free instant pudding mix	1 pkg. (4-serving)
2 c.	low-fat milk	500 mL
1 T.	fresh lemon juice	15 mL
2 t.	grated lemon rind	10 mL
1	egg yolk, slightly beaten	1

Combine pudding mix, milk, lemon juice, and lemon rind in a nonstick saucepan. Cook and stir until mixture just comes to a boil. Stir a small amount of pudding mixture into beaten egg; then return to saucepan. Continue cooking until mixture comes to full boil. Remove from heat. Pour into large dessert dish or four smaller dishes or margarita glasses.

Yield: 4 servings
Exchange, 1 serving: 1 low-fat milk
Calories, 1 serving: 100
Carbohydrates, 1 serving: 12 g

Coconut Custard

1 pkg. (4-serving)	vanilla-flavored sugar-free instant pudding mix	1 pkg. (4-serving)
2 c.	low-fat milk	500 mL
⅔ c.	unsweetened coconut flakes, toasted	180 mL
1	egg yolk, slightly beaten	1

Combine pudding mix, milk, and ½ c. (125 mL) of the toasted coconut in a saucepan. Cook and stir until mixture just comes to a boil. Pour a small amount of mixture into beaten egg yolk; then return to saucepan. Cook until mixture comes to a full boil. Cover with wax paper and allow to cool slightly. Spoon into six dessert dishes. Top with remaining toasted coconut. Refrigerate to chill thoroughly.

Yield: 6 servings
Exchange, 1 serving: ½ low-fat milk, 1 fat
Calories, 1 serving: 110
Carbohydrates, 1 serving: 9 g

True Chocolate Custard

2 c.	skim milk	500 mL
1 T.	vegetable oil	15 mL
1 t.	vanilla extract	5 mL
2 oz.	semisweet chocolate, chopped	57 g
6	egg yolks	6
2 T.	granulated fructose	30 mL

Combine skim milk, vegetable oil, and vanilla in a saucepan. Bring to a simmer. Remove from heat; stir in chocolate until melted and mixture is smooth. Whisk egg yolks and fructose in a medium bowl. Very slowly whisk egg yolk mixture into hot chocolate. Cool to room temperature, stirring occasionally. Position a rack in the middle of the oven. Preheat oven to 300 °F (150 °C). Place six custard cups in a shallow baking pan. Evenly divide the chocolate mixture between the cups. Fill baking pan with enough hot water to come halfway up the sides of the custard cups. Bake until custards are just set, about 35 to 40 minutes. Cool or serve warm.

Yield: 6 servings
Exchange, 1 serving: 1 skim milk, 1 fat
Calories, 1 serving: 150
Carbohydrates, 1 serving: 11 g

Hot Peach Pudding

1 lb.	dried peaches	454 g
3 c.	water	750 mL
1 pkg.	vanilla-flavored sugar-free instant	1 pkg.
(4-serving)	pudding mix	(4-serving)

Rinse peaches under cool water. Combine peaches and 3 c. (750 mL) of the water in a saucepan. Cook until tender; then remove peaches, cool, and cut into pieces. Continue cooking peach water until reduced to about 1 c. (250 mL); then return peaches to pan. Meanwhile, prepare pudding mix as directed on package. Allow to thicken for 10 minutes. Add hot peaches and peach juice. Serve hot.

Yield: 4 servings
Exchange, 1 serving: 1 fruit
Calories, 1 serving: 58
Carbohydrates, 1 serving: 12 g

Coffee Pudding

1 pkg.	vanilla-flavored sugar-free instant	1 pkg.
(4-serving)	pudding mix	(4-serving)
1 c.	skim milk, scalded and cooled	250 mL
1 c.	cool strong coffee	250 mL
4 T.	prepared nondairy whipped topping	60 mL

Combine all ingredients except whipped topping in saucepan. Stir to blend. Cook and stir over medium heat until mixture comes to full boil. Let boil for 2 minutes; cool slightly. Pour into four dessert glasses. Just before serving, top each glass with 1 T. (15 mL) of nondairy whipped topping.

Yield: 4 servings
Exchange, 1 serving: ¾ skim milk
Calories, 1 serving: 43
Carbohydrates, 1 serving: 8 g

Favorite Chocolate Mousse

2 c.	cold skim milk	500 mL
2 T.	all-purpose flour	30 mL
4 t.	granulated fructose	20 mL
2	eggs, separated	2
¼ c.	semisweet chocolate chips	60 mL

Combine cold milk, flour, and fructose in a 1½-qt. (1½-L) microwave safe bowl. Whisk to completely dissolve the flour and fructose. Microwave, uncovered, on HIGH for 4 minutes. Meanwhile, beat egg yolks with a small whisk or fork. Pour and mix a small amount of the hot milk-pudding mixture into the egg yolk. Then stir the egg yolk mixture into the remaining hot pudding. Return to the microwave and cook on HIGH for 2 minutes, stirring after 1 minute. Remove from microwave and add chocolate chips. Stir until chips are completely melted and mixture is smooth. Refrigerate until completely chilled and set. (You can do the first part in the morning and the second part just before dinner.) Second part: Beat egg whites until stiff. (Egg whites beat up faster when they are at room temperature.) Fold a small amount of the chocolate pudding into the egg whites. Fold egg white mixture into remaining chocolate pudding. Spoon into six wine glasses. Chill until ready to serve.

Yield: 6 servings
Exchange, 1 serving: 1 low-fat milk
Calories, 1 serving: 110
Carbohydrates, 1 serving: 12 g

Orange Cream Custard

1 pkg.	vanilla-flavored sugar-free instant	1 pkg.
(4-serving)	pudding mix	(4-serving)
1 c.	low-fat milk	250 mL
1 c.	orange juice	250 mL
1	egg, separated	1
4	orange sections	4

Combine pudding mix, milk, and orange juice in a saucepan. Cook and stir over medium heat just until mixture comes to a boil. Meanwhile, slightly beat the egg yolk. Pour a small amount of pudding mixture into the egg yolk, stir, and return mixture to saucepan. Continue cooking until mixture comes to a full boil. Remove from heat, cover with wax paper, and cool slightly. Spoon into four dessert glasses. Refrigerate and chill until firm. Beat egg white until stiff. Just before serving, garnish with whipped egg white and orange section.

Yield: 4 servings
Exchange, 1 serving: 1 low-fat milk, ⅓ fat
Calories, 1 serving: 126
Carbohydrates, 1 serving: 16 g

Maple Raisin Pudding

½ c.	raisins	125 mL
2 c.	water	500 mL
¼ t.	maple flavoring	1 mL
1 pkg.	vanilla-flavored sugar-free instant	1 pkg.
(4-serving)	pudding mix	(4-serving)
4 T.	prepared nondairy whipped topping	60 mL

Combine raisins and water in a nonstick saucepan. Bring to a boil. Remove from heat; cool to room temperature. Stir in maple flavoring. Drain raisin water into a bowl. Add pudding mix, stirring as directed on package. Spoon into dessert dishes or wine glasses in three layers: raisins, maple pudding, and a dab of dairy topping.

Yield: 4 servings
Exchange, 1 serving: 1¼ fruit
Calories, 1 serving: 83
Carbohydrates, 1 serving: 20 g

Chocolate Polka-Dot Pudding

1 pkg.	chocolate-flavored sugar-free instant	1 pkg.
(4-serving)	pudding mix	(4-serving)
¼ c.	mini–chocolate chips	60 mL

Make pudding mix as directed on package. Chill until set. Fold in chocolate chips. Spoon into dessert dishes.

Yield: 4 servings
Exchange, 1 serving: 1 skim milk, 1 fat
Calories, 1 serving: 135
Carbohydrates, 1 serving: 17 g

Creamy Pumpkin Pudding

1 c.	pureed pumpkin	250 mL
¾ c.	water	190 mL
1 pkg.	butterscotch-flavored sugar-free	1 pkg.
(4-serving)	instant pudding mix	(4-serving)

Combine pumpkin and water in a saucepan or microwave bowl. Heat on HIGH until boiling. Remove from heat and chill thoroughly. Whisk or beat in pudding mix. Spoon into four dessert dishes.

Yield: 4 servings
Exchange, 1 serving: 1 fruit
Calories, 1 serving: 50
Carbohydrates, 1 serving: 13 g

Prune Whip

2 jars (4-oz.)	baby prunes	2 jars (113-g)
2 t.	lemon juice	10 mL
2	egg whites	2
dash	salt	dash
¼ c.	granulated sugar replacement	60 mL

Combine strained prunes and lemon juice in a small bowl; stir to mix. Beat the egg whites and salt to soft peaks. Gradually add the sugar replacement; beat to stiff peaks. Fold prune mixture into stiffly beaten egg whites. Spoon into four sherbet or dessert glasses. Chill.

Yield: 4 servings
Exchange, 1 serving: 1 fruit
Calories, 1 serving: 56
Carbohydrates, 1 serving: 13 g

Pineapple Bread Pudding

9-oz. can	crushed pineapple, in juice	256-g can
2 c.	soft white-bread crumbs	500 mL
2 c.	skim milk	500 mL
¼ t.	salt	1 mL
2	eggs, beaten	2
2 T.	granulated fructose	30 mL

Drain pineapple juice into a measuring cup; add enough water to the juice to make ¼ c. (60 mL) of liquid. Combine crushed pineapple, pineapple liquid, and remaining ingredients in a large bowl. Fold to blend. Pour into a 1½-qt. (1½-L) baking dish. Bake at 325 °F (165 °C) for about 45 minutes or until set.

Yield: 6 servings
Exchange, 1 serving: ½ bread, 1 fruit, ⅓ skim milk
Calories, 1 serving: 128
Carbohydrates, 1 serving: 19 g

Cup o' Java Pudding

1 pkg.	vanilla-flavored sugar-free instant	1 pkg.
(4-serving)	pudding mix	(4-serving)
2 c.	low-fat milk	500 mL
2 t.	instant coffee powder	10 mL
1	egg white, stiffly beaten	1
1 c.	prepared nondairy whipped topping	250 mL

Combine pudding mix and coffee powder in a saucepan. Add milk and prepare pudding mix as directed on package. Remove from heat. Slowly pour hot pudding over stiffly beaten egg white. Fold slightly. Cover and chill. To serve: Alternate layers of pudding mix and nondairy whipped topping in four wine, parfait, or dessert glasses.

Yield: 4 servings
Exchange, 1 serving: 1 bread
Calories, 1 serving: 114
Carbohydrates, 1 serving: 13 g

Wild Blueberry Pudding

1 pkg.	vanilla-flavored sugar-free instant	1 pkg.
(4-serving)	pudding mix	(4-serving)
2 c.	cold low-fat milk	500 mL
½ c.	all-natural wild blueberry preserves	125 mL

Combine ingredients in a bowl. Beat until well blended, about 1 or 2 minutes. Spoon into dessert glasses. Refrigerate until ready to serve.

Yield: 6 servings
Exchange, 1 serving: 1 bread
Calories, 1 serving: 98
Carbohydrates, 1 serving: 14 g

Noodle-Apple Chocolate Pudding

1 pkg.	chocolate fudge–flavored sugar-free	1 pkg.
(4-serving)	instant pudding mix	(4-serving)
1 c.	cooked wide noodles	250 mL
1	red Delicious apple, peeled and grated	1
¼ c.	chopped almonds	60 mL
¼ t.	cinnamon	1 mL

Prepare pudding as directed on package. Refrigerate to set. Fold in remaining ingredients. Spoon into six dessert glasses. Refrigerate until ready to serve.

Yield: 6 servings
Exchange, 1 serving: ½ low-fat milk, 1 fat
Calories, 1 serving: 102
Carbohydrates, 1 serving: 12 g

Quick Vanilla Rice Pudding

1 pkg.	vanilla-flavored sugar-free	1 pkg.
(4-serving)	instant pudding mix	(4-serving)
2 c.	skim milk	500 mL
1 c.	chilled cooked instant rice	250 mL

Combine vanilla pudding mix and skim milk in a bowl or shaker bottle and prepare as directed on package. Chill to allow to set completely. Fold cooked rice into pudding. Spoon into six dessert glasses. Refrigerate.

Yield: 6 servings
Exchange, 1 serving: 1 bread
Calories, 1 serving: 81
Carbohydrates, 1 serving: 15 g

Rice Pudding with Strawberry Topping

1 recipe	"Quick Vanilla Rice Pudding," prepared (above)	1 recipe
3 c.	strawberries, washed and hulled	750 mL
1 T.	granulated sugar replacement	15 mL
	mint leaves (optional)	

Place strawberries and sugar replacement in a blender or food processor. Process into a puree. Spoon strawberry topping over rice pudding just before serving. Garnish with mint leaves if desired.

Yield: 6 servings
Exchange, 1 serving: 1 bread, ½ fruit
Calories, 1 serving: 110
Carbohydrates, 1 serving: 21 g

Chocolate-Fudge Rice Pudding

1 pkg.	chocolate fudge–flavored sugar-free	1 pkg.
(4-serving)	instant pudding mix	(4-serving)
1½ c.	cold cooked rice	325 mL
6 sprigs	mint leaves (optional)	6 sprigs

Prepare pudding as directed on package. Chill to completely set. Fold in cooked rice. Spoon into six dessert glasses. Refrigerate to keep cold. Just before serving, garnish with mint leaves.

Yield: 6 servings
Exchange, 1 serving: ⅔ bread, ½ low-fat milk
Calories, 1 serving: 116
Carbohydrates, 1 serving: 21 g

Maple Rice Pudding

8 oz.	nonfat vanilla yogurt	240 g
¼ c.	Cary's Sugar-Free Maple-Flavored Syrup	60 mL
1 t.	vanilla extract	5 mL
12	thin apple slices	12
1 T.	lemon juice	15 mL
2 c.	chilled cooked instant rice	500 mL

Combine yogurt, maple syrup, and vanilla extract in a bowl. Stir to blend. Refrigerate until ready to serve. Sprinkle apple slices with lemon juice. Wrap tightly with plastic wrap. Refrigerate until ready to serve. Just before serving, fold chilled cooked rice into yogurt mixture. Spoon into six wine or dessert glasses. Garnish each glass with two apple slices.

Yield: 6 servings
Exchange, 1 serving: 1 bread, ¼ skim milk
Calories, 1 serving: 95
Carbohydrates, 1 serving: 19 g

Crisps & Cobblers

For many people, the words "crisps," "cobblers," and "Betties" conjure up thoughts of home. They are simple desserts made with nothing more than fruit and a crust or crumb topping. Almost every fruit can be used in either a crisp or a cobbler. These creations were developed by our great-great-great-grandmothers. They were originally made from whatever was in the kitchen or growing in the garden at the time. Therefore, we basically have the same dessert with many different kinds of fruit (fresh or dried), topped or bottomed (or both) with a crust.

Ginger Pear Crumble

30	gingersnaps	30
30-oz. can	pear halves, in juice	855-g can
1 T.	lemon juice	15 mL
½ t.	ground cinnamon	2 mL
¼ t.	salt	1 mL
¼ t.	ground nutmeg	1 mL

Using a food processor or blender, grind the gingersnaps into crumbs. Arrange half of the gingersnap crumbs on the bottom of a 1½-qt. (1½-L) baking dish that has been sprayed with vegetable oil. Drain pears, reserving ¼ c. (60 mL) of the liquid. Place pears on the crumbs. Add lemon juice to the reserved pear liquid and sprinkle over pears. Mix cinnamon, salt, and nutmeg together. Sprinkle on top of pears. Top with remaining gingersnap crumbs. Bake at 350 °F (175 °C) for about 25 minutes.

Yield: 6 servings
Exchange, 1 serving: ½ bread, ⅓ fruit
Calories, 1 serving: 160
Carbohydrates, 1 serving: 21 g

Blueberry Crisp

1 qt.	frozen or fresh blueberries	1 L
2 T.	granulated fructose	30 mL
2 T.	lemon juice	30 mL
2 T.	water	30 mL

Topping

1 c.	quick-cooking oatmeal	250 mL
¼ c.	all-purpose flour	60 mL
¼ c.	chopped walnuts	60 mL
3 T.	granulated fructose	45 mL
⅓ c.	firm margarine	90 mL

Place the blueberries in a shallow 1½-qt. (1½-L) baking dish. Sprinkle with 2 T. (30 mL) of the fructose, lemon juice, and water. Stir to mix evenly. Combine oatmeal, flour, walnuts, and 3 T. (45 mL) of the fructose in a small bowl. Cut margarine into mixture or rub with the fingers until mixture becomes coarse crumbs. Sprinkle evenly over the top of the blueberry mixture. Bake at 350 °F (175 °C) uncovered for 30 to 40 minutes or until topping is browned and berries are tender. Serve hot or cold.

Yield: 8 servings
Exchange, 1 serving: 1 fruit, ⅓ bread, 2 fat
Calories, 1 serving: 187
Carbohydrates, 1 serving: 21 g

Delicious Apple Crisp

3 medium	golden Delicious apples	3 medium
2 medium	red Delicious apples	2 medium
⅓ c.	white grape juice	90 mL

Topping

1 c.	all-purpose flour	250 mL
3 T.	granulated sugar replacement	45 mL
¾ t.	ground cinnamon	4 mL
¼ t.	salt	1 mL
¼ c.	firm margarine	60 mL

Core the apples and cut them into ½-in.-(1.25-cm-) thick slices. (Skin is left on for color.) Distribute apple slices evenly on the bottom of a well-greased

7 × 11 in. (17 × 27 cm) baking pan. Pour grape juice over the apple slices. In a small bowl, combine flour, sugar replacement, cinnamon, and salt. Cut the margarine into the flour mixture or rub with the fingers until the mixture becomes coarse crumbs. Sprinkle evenly over the apples. Bake at 375 °F (190 °C) for 30 to 35 minutes or until topping is browned and apples are tender. Serve hot or cold.

Yield: 8 servings
Exchange, 1 serving: 1 fruit, ⅔ bread, 1 fat
Calories, 1 serving: 161
Carbohydrates, 1 serving: 25 g

Pear and Mandarin Orange Crisp

1-lb. can	pear halves in juice	454-g can
15-oz. can	mandarin orange sections in water	425-g can
2 t.	granulated fructose	10 mL
1 t.	cornstarch	5 mL

Topping

6	graham cracker squares	6
⅓ c.	all-purpose flour	90 mL
1 t.	granulated fructose	5 mL
1 t.	vanilla extract	5 mL
3 T.	firm margarine	45 mL

Drain ½ c. (125 mL) of the pear juice from the can into a measuring cup; reserve. Drain the pears, and arrange pear halves in the bottom of a 1-qt. (1-L) well-greased baking dish. Drain the mandarin oranges, and pour orange sections over the pear halves. Add the 2 t. (10 mL) of fructose and the cornstarch to the reserved pear juice; stir to dissolve. Pour over fruit in baking dish. Crush graham crackers. Combine graham cracker crumbs, flour, 1 t. (5 mL) of the fructose, and vanilla in a small bowl. Cut the margarine into the flour mixture or rub with the fingers until the mixture becomes coarse crumbs. Sprinkle evenly over the fruit. Bake at 350 °F (175 °C) for 30 to 35 minutes or until topping is browned. Serve hot or cold.

Yield: 8 servings
Exchange, 1 serving: ⅔ fruit, ½ bread, 1 fat
Calories, 1 serving: 119
Carbohydrates, 1 serving: 18 g

Royal Anne Cherry Coconut Crisp

16-oz. can	Royal Anne cherries in water	454-g can
1 t.	lemon juice	5 mL
2 t.	water	10 mL
1 T.	granulated fructose	15 mL
1 t.	ground nutmeg	5 mL

Topping

½ c.	quick-cooking oatmeal	125 mL
2 T.	all-purpose flour	30 mL
¼ c.	unsweetened coconut	60 mL
2 T.	granulated fructose	30 mL
¼ c.	firm margarine	60 mL

Drain cherries. Divide evenly between four oven-proof serving dishes. Sprinkle with lemon juice and water. Combine 1 T. (15 mL) of the fructose and the nutmeg; sprinkle evenly over the four servings. Combine oatmeal, flour, coconut, and 2 T. (30 mL) of the fructose in a bowl. Cut margarine into mixture, forming coarse crumbs. Sprinkle evenly over the top of cherries. Bake at 350 °F (175 °C) for 20 to 30 minutes or until topping is browned. Serve hot or cold.

Yield: 4 servings
Exchange, 1 serving: 1 fruit, 1 fat
Calories, 1 serving: 120
Carbohydrates, 1 serving: 18 g

Banana Crisp on a Stick

1 pkg. (4-serving)	sugar-free orange gelatin	1 pkg. (4-serving)
¼ c.	corn flakes	60 mL
1 t.	granulated fructose	5 mL
1	large banana	1

Prepare gelatin as directed on package. Allow to cool until thick but not set. Crush corn flakes and spread on a small plate. Sprinkle with fructose. Peel banana and cut in half horizontally. Place each half on the end of a wooden popsicle or lollipop stick. Dip banana halves into thickened gelatin. Then roll each banana half in the corn-flake crumbs. Press crumbs lightly into sides of banana. Cool or eat immediately. (You will not use all of the gelatin.) Children love 'em.

Yield: 2 servings
Exchange, 1 serving: 1 fruit, ¼ bread
Calories, 1 serving: 76
Carbohydrates, 1 serving: 20 g

Apple Cranberry Shortcake

Shortcake

3 c.	biscuit mix	750 mL
3 T.	firm shortening	45 mL
1	egg	1
⅔ c.	skim milk	180 mL
1 T.	margarine, melted	15 mL

Sauce

1 qt.	apples, peeled and thinly sliced	1 L
1 c.	cranberries	250 mL
¼ c.	water	60 mL
⅓ c.	granulated brown-sugar replacement	90 mL
¼ c.	granulated fructose	60 mL
1 t.	caramel flavoring	5 mL
dash	salt	dash

Combine biscuit mix and shortening in a medium-sized bowl. Cut shortening into mix to form coarse crumbs. Combine egg and skim milk in a bowl. Beat slightly to blend. Pour into biscuit mix. Stir to moisten dry ingredients. Divide dough in half. Pat half of the dough on the bottom of a 9-in. (23-cm) layer cake pan. Brush with the melted margarine. Roll out remaining dough and place on top of dough in cake pan. Bake at 425 °F (220 °C) for 20 to 25 minutes. Meanwhile, combine ingredients for sauce in a heavy nonstick saucepan. Bring to a boil and boil until apple slices are tender. Turn shortcake out onto serving tray. Remove top layer of cake. Fill bottom layer with half of the apple cranberry sauce. Return top to cake, and spoon remaining sauce over top. To serve: Cut cake into nine wedges.

Yield: 9 servings
Exchange, 1 serving: 1⅓ bread, 1 fruit, 1½ fat
Calories, 1 serving: 314
Carbohydrates, 1 serving: 36 g

Fruit Cobblers

1 tube	ready-to-bake biscuits	1 tube
(10 count)		(10 count)

Prepare any of the fruit fillings below. Pour filling into an 8-in. (20-cm) round baking pan. Lay biscuits on top of filling. Bake at 400 °F (200 °C) for 20 to 25 minutes. Serve warm or chilled.

Tart Cherry Filling

1-lb. 4-oz. can	pitted tart cherries (water packed)	545-g can
¼ c.	granulated fructose	60 mL
1 T.	quick-cooking tapioca	15 mL
	red food coloring (optional)	

Do not drain the cherries. Combine ingredients in a saucepan. Cook and stir until boiling and slightly thickened.

Yield: 10 servings
Exchange, 1 serving tart cherries: 1 bread, ⅓ fruit
Calories, 1 serving tart cherries: 90
Carbohydrates, 1 serving tart cherries: 20 g

Fresh Peach Filling

1½ T.	cornstarch	23 mL
¼ c.	granulated sugar replacement	60 mL
¼ t.	ground nutmeg	1 mL
½ c.	water	125 mL
1 qt.	peaches, peeled and sliced	1 L
1 T.	lemon juice	15 mL

Combine cornstarch, sugar replacement, nutmeg, and water in a saucepan. Cook and stir until thickened. Add sliced peaches and lemon juice. Cook 5 minutes longer.

Yield: 10 servings
Exchange, 1 serving fresh peaches: 1 bread, ½ fruit
Calories, 1 serving fresh peaches: 103
Carbohydrates, 1 serving fresh peaches: 25 g

Apple Filling

1-lb. 4-oz. can	Musselman's sliced apples	567-g can
¼ c.	water	60 mL
1½ T.	cornstarch	23 mL
2 T.	granulated fructose	30 mL

| ½ t. | ground cinnamon | 2 mL |
| ¼ t. | ground nutmeg | 1 mL |

Combine all ingredients in a saucepan. Stir to mix. Cook and stir until hot.

Yield: 10 servings
Exchange, 1 serving sliced apples: 1 bread, ⅓ fruit
Calories, 1 serving sliced apples: 92
Carbohydrates, 1 serving sliced apples: 21 g

Rhubarb Cobbler

1 lb.	fresh or frozen rhubarb	500 g
	(cut in 1-in. (2.5-cm) pieces)	
½ c.	granulated fructose	125 mL
¼ c.	water	60 mL
⅔ c.	all-purpose flour	180 mL
⅓ c.	whole-wheat pastry flour	90 mL
1½ t.	baking powder	7 mL
dash	salt	dash
2 T.	firm margarine	30 mL
½ c.	skim milk	125 mL

Place rhubarb in a bowl. Sprinkle with fructose and water. Toss to completely coat. Place in a 1½-qt. (1½-L) well-greased baking dish. Combine all-purpose flour, wheat flour, baking powder, and salt in a bowl. Cut the firm margarine into the flour mixture until mixture becomes coarse crumbs. Stir in the skim milk. Drop the cobbler batter in eight equal spoonfuls on top of rhubarb. Bake at 375 °F (190 °C) for 25 to 30 minutes or until batter is golden brown and rhubarb is tender.

Yield: 8 servings
Exchange, 1 serving: 1 bread, ½ fat
Calories, 1 serving: 107
Carbohydrates, 1 serving: 18 g

Cakes

Making a cake today is a snap. There aren't any real secrets in using a cake mix. And when you add a few of your own flavors, those unimaginative cake mixes become truly special desserts. If you are uncertain about what flavors to add, check with your family and friends. Everyone has a favorite.

I have included a cake from a cake mix in which you will find yeast used. You can use yeast in any of the other cakes as well. The yeast helps the cake to rise, and the cake will be lighter and fill the pan.

One benefit of baking a cake is that it freezes. After baking and cooling, cut the cake into individual-serving slices. Wrap each slice in a piece of plastic wrap, place in a freezer container, and freeze. Just go to your freezer the next time you need a dessert.

Easy Pineapple Cake

| 8-oz. pkg. | sugar-free yellow cake mix | 226-g pkg. |
| 2/3 c. | unsweetened pineapple juice | 180 mL |

Combine cake mix and half of the pineapple juice in a mixing bowl. Beat on HIGH for 3 minutes. Add remaining juice and continue beating for 3 more minutes. Transfer to an 8-in. (20-cm) wax-paper–lined or greased-and-floured cake pan. Bake at 375 °F (190 °C) for 25 minutes or until tester inserted in middle comes out clean.

Yield: 10 servings
Exchange, 1 serving: 1 bread, ½ fruit, ½ fat
Calories, 1 serving: 104
Carbohydrates, 1 serving: 20 g

Fast Spice Cake

8-oz. pkg.	sugar-free lemon cake mix	226-g pkg.
1 t.	ground cinnamon	5 mL
½ t.	ground nutmeg	2 mL
¼ t.	ground allspice	1 mL

| ¼ t. | ground cloves | 1 mL |
| ⅔ c. | water | 180 mL |

Place cake mix in mixing bowl. Add spices to dry ingredients. Add ⅓ c. (90 mL) of the water to the mixture. Beat on HIGH for 3 minutes. Add remaining water and continue beating for 3 more minutes. Transfer to an 8-in. (20-cm) wax-paper–lined or greased-and-floured cake pan. Bake at 375 °F (190 °C) for 25 minutes or until tester inserted in middle comes out clean.

Yield: 10 servings
Exchange, 1 serving: 1 bread, ½ fat
Calories, 1 serving: 96
Carbohydrates, 1 serving: 16 g

Lemon Lime Creme Cake

3	egg whites	3
dash	salt	dash
1	lime	1
8-oz. pkg.	sugar-free yellow cake mix	226-g pkg.
2 c.	prepared nondairy whipped topping	500 mL

Beat egg whites and salt until stiff. Wash and finely grate the peel of the lime to about 2 t. (30 mL). Soften lime and squeeze out the juice. Pour lime juice into a measuring cup; add enough water to make ⅔ c. (180 mL) of liquid. Combine cake mix, grated lime peel, and ⅓ c. (90 mL) of the liquid in a mixing bowl. Beat on HIGH for 3 minutes. Add remaining juice and continue beating for 3 more minutes. Fold 1 c. (250 mL) of the stiffly beaten egg white into the cake batter. Gently fold in remaining egg whites. Fit a piece of wax paper on the bottom of an 8-in. (20-cm) cake pan. Transfer cake batter to pan. Bake at 375 °F (190 °C) for 25 minutes or until tester inserted in middle comes out clean. Cool in the pan for about 10 minutes; then transfer cake to rack. Remove wax paper. Cool completely. Cut cake in half horizontally. Remove top. Transfer bottom layer of cake to plate. Spread 1 c. (250 mL) of the nondairy whipped topping on bottom layer. Cover with top layer of cake. Frost top layer with remaining whipped topping. Chill or serve immediately.

Yield: 10 servings
Exchange, 1 serving: 1 bread, 1 fat
Calories, 1 serving: 126
Carbohydrates, 1 serving: 19 g

Orange Flower Cake

1	orange	1
8-oz. pkg.	sugar-free yellow cake mix	226-g pkg.
⅔ c.	orange juice	180 mL
1 c.	prepared nondairy whipped topping	250 mL

Wash and finely grate 1 T. (15 mL) of orange peel. Peel and remove white membrane from the orange. Carefully divide the orange into segments; remove outer membrane from each segment. Set aside. Combine cake mix, grated orange peel, and ⅓ c. (90 mL) of the orange juice in a mixing bowl. Beat on HIGH for 3 minutes. Add remaining juice and continue beating for 3 more minutes. Transfer to an 8-in. (20-cm) wax-paper–lined or greased-and-floured cake pan. Bake at 375 °F (190 °C) for 25 minutes or until tester inserted in middle comes out clean. Cool in the pan for about 10 minutes; then transfer cake to rack. Cool completely. Transfer cake to decorative plate. Frost top of cake with nondairy whipped topping. Place orange segments in flower design on the whipped topping. Chill or serve immediately.

Yield: 10 servings
Exchange, 1 serving: 1 bread, ¼ fruit, ½ fat
Calories, 1 serving: 120
Carbohydrates, 1 serving: 19 g

Mocha Cake

8-oz. pkg.	sugar-free chocolate cake mix	226-g pkg.
½ t.	ground cinnamon	2 mL
⅔ c.	strong coffee	180 mL

Place cake mix in mixing bowl. Add cinnamon to cake mix. Add ⅓ c. (90 mL) of the coffee to the mixture. Beat on HIGH for 3 minutes. Add remaining coffee and continue beating for 3 more minutes. Transfer to an 8-in. (20-cm) wax-paper–lined or greased-and-floured cake pan. Bake at 375 °F (190 °C) for 25 minutes or until tester inserted in middle comes out clean. Cool cake in pan for about 10 minutes. Remove from pan. Serve warm, or cool completely.

Yield: 10 servings
Exchange, 1 serving: 1 bread, ½ fat
Calories, 1 serving: 98
Carbohydrates, 1 serving: 16 g

Chocolate Chocolate Mint Cake

8-oz. pkg.	sugar-free chocolate cake mix	226-g pkg.
⅔ c.	water	180 mL
½ t.	mint flavoring	2 mL
½ c.	mini–chocolate mint chips	125 mL
2	egg whites, stiffly beaten	2

Combine cake mix, water, and mint flavoring in a mixing bowl. Beat on MEDIUM for 5 to 6 minutes or until batter is thick and creamy. Add chips. Fold in stiffly beaten egg whites. Transfer to a wax-paper–lined or greased-and-floured 8-in. (20-cm) round cake pan. Bake at 350 °F (175 °C) for 20 to 25 minutes or until tester inserted in middle comes out clean. Cool in the pan for about 10 minutes; then transfer cake to rack. Cool completely.

Yield: 10 servings
Exchange, 1 serving: 1 bread, 1½ fat
Calories, 1 serving: 133
Carbohydrates, 1 serving: 21 g

Peach Crunch Pie Cake

8-oz. pkg.	sugar-free white cake mix	226-g pkg.
1	egg white	1
⅔ c.	water	180 mL
½ t.	vanilla extract	2 mL
2	peaches, peeled and thinly sliced	2
½ c.	corn flakes	125 mL

Combine cake mix, egg white, water, and vanilla extract in a mixing bowl. Beat on MEDIUM for 5 to 6 minutes or until batter is thick and creamy. Transfer to a greased-and-floured 9-in. (23-cm) pie pan. Lay the thin slices of peaches around the edge of the cake batter in a circular fashion. Crush corn flakes; sprinkle evenly on top of peach slices and batter. Bake at 350 °F (175 °C) for 15 to 20 minutes or until tester inserted in middle comes out clean. Cool and serve from pie pan.

Yield: 10 servings
Exchange, 1 serving: 1 bread, ½ fat
Calories, 1 serving: 97
Carbohydrates, 1 serving: 18 g

Quick Marble Cake

| 8-oz. pkg. | sugar-free chocolate cake mix | 226-g pkg. |
| 8-oz. pkg. | sugar-free white cake mix | 226-g pkg. |

Prepare cake mixes as directed on package in two separate bowls. Wax-paper–line or lightly grease and flour the sides and bottom of a 9-in.- (23-cm-) square cake pan. Drop batter by tablespoons into the pan, alternating chocolate and white batters. Bake at 350 °F (175 °C) for 25 to 35 minutes or until tester inserted in middle comes out clean. Cool in the pan for about 10 minutes; then transfer cake to rack. Cool completely. Cut cake into 20 servings.

Yield: 20 servings
Exchange, 1 serving: 1 bread, ½ fat
Calories, 1 serving: 97
Carbohydrates, 1 serving: 16 g

Sweet Potato Cake

1	egg	1
6-oz. jar	sweet potatoes, baby	170-g jar
½ t.	cinnamon	2 mL
8-oz. pkg.	sugar-free pound cake mix	226-g pkg.
⅔ c.	water	180 mL

Beat egg in a medium-sized mixing bowl until light lemon colored and fluffy. Beat in sweet potatoes and cinnamon. Add cake mix and water alternately in small amounts, beating well after each addition. Beat a minute more. Pour into wax-paper–lined or greased-and-floured 8 × 4 × 2 in. (20 × 10 × 5 cm) loaf pan, and bake at 350 °F (175 °C) for 45 to 50 minutes. Cool cake in pan for 10 minutes. Turn cake out onto rack and cool completely or serve warm.

Yield: 10 servings
Exchange, 1 serving: 1 bread, ½ fat
Calories, 1 serving: 104
Carbohydrates, 1 serving: 18 g

Carrot Cake with Raisins and Nuts

⅓ c.	raisins	90 mL
2 T.	bourbon	30 mL
1	egg	1

1	egg white	1
6-oz. jar	baby carrots	170-g jar
⅓ c.	walnuts	90 mL
8-oz. pkg.	sugar-free pound cake mix	226-g pkg.
½ t.	ground cinnamon	2 mL
¼ t.	ground nutmeg	1 mL
¼ t.	ground allspice	1 mL
⅔ c.	water	180 mL

Chop or snip raisins into about thirds; place in a small bowl and sprinkle with bourbon. Allow to rest until needed. Beat egg and egg white in a medium-sized mixing bowl until light lemon colored and fluffy. Beat in carrots. Stir in bourboned raisins and walnuts. Add spices to cake mix and stir slightly to mix. Add spiced cake mix and water alternately in small amounts to beaten-egg mixture, beating well after each addition. Beat a minute more. Transfer to a wax-paper–lined or greased-and-floured 9-in.- (23-cm-) square cake pan. Bake at 375 °F (190 °C) for 40 to 50 minutes or until tester inserted in middle comes out clean. Cool in the pan for about 10 minutes; then transfer cake to rack. Cool completely. Cut cake into 20 servings.

Yield: 20 servings
Exchange, 1 serving: 1 bread, ¼ fruit, 1 fat
Calories, 1 serving: 144
Carbohydrates, 1 serving: 21 g

Citrus Devil's Food Cake

8-oz. pkg.	sugar-free chocolate cake mix	226-g pkg.
1	egg white	1
⅔ c.	grapefruit juice	180 mL

Combine cake mix and egg white in a mixing bowl. Add grapefruit juice. Beat on LOW for 1 minute. Continue beating on HIGH 5 minutes more or until batter is thick and very creamy. Transfer to a wax-paper–lined or greased-and-floured 8-in. round cake pan. Bake at 350 °F (175 °C) for 20 to 25 minutes. Cool for 10 minutes in the pan. Turn cake out onto a cooling rack; cool completely.

Yield: 10 servings
Exchange, 1 serving: 1 bread, ½ fat
Calories, 1 serving: 91
Carbohydrates, 1 serving: 17 g

Heavenly Blueberry Cake

2 pkgs. (8-oz.)	sugar-free yellow cake mix	2 pkgs. (226-g)
2 env.	unflavored gelatin	2 env.
½ c.	cold water	125 mL
2 pkgs. (1-lb.)	Flavorland frozen blueberries, thawed	2 pkgs. (454-g)
2 c.	prepared nondairy whipped topping mint sprigs	500 mL

Prepare cake mixes together as directed on package; bake together in one 8-in.- (20-cm-) square pan, with the bottom lined with wax paper. Cool cake slightly in pan. Carefully release cake from sides of pan by sliding a sharp knife between cake and sides of pan. Transfer to rack, remove wax paper, and cool completely. Cut cake into ¼-in. (8-mm) slices. Then cut each slice in half. Lightly grease the 9-in. (23-cm) springform, or loose bottom, pan. Line bottom and sides of springform pan with cake slices. Soften gelatin in ½ c. (125 mL) of cold water. Heat slightly either in a microwave or on top of the stove. Stir to completely dissolve gelatin. Place thawed blueberries and any juice in a mixing bowl, and slightly crush some of the berries. Stir in softened gelatin and nondairy whipped topping. Pour about a fourth of the berry mixture into the cake-lined pan. Arrange about a third of the remaining cake pieces and crumbs over the berry mixture. Repeat with the next two layers, ending with a layer of the berry mixture. Chill overnight or until completely set. Remove sides of springform, or loose bottom, pan. Place cake with pan bottom on dessert platter. Garnish plate and cake with mint sprigs. Chill until serving time.

Yield: 20 servings
Exchange, 1 serving: 1 bread, ½ fruit, ½ fat
Calories, 1 serving: 144
Carbohydrates, 1 serving: 25 g

So Good Chocolate Cake

8-oz. pkg.	sugar-free chocolate cake mix	226-g pkg.
1 T.	unsweetened cocoa powder	15 mL
1	egg white	1
⅔ c.	spiced-tomato vegetable juice	180 mL

Combine cake mix, cocoa, and egg white in a mixing bowl. Add vegetable juice. Stir to mix. Beat on HIGH 5 to 6 minutes more or until batter is thick and very creamy. Transfer to a greased-and-floured 8-in. round cake pan.

Bake at 350 °F (175 °C) for 20 to 25 minutes. Cool for 10 minutes in the pan. Turn cake out onto a serving plate. Serve warm.

Yield: 10 servings
Exchange, 1 serving: 1 bread, ½ fat
Calories, 1 serving: 92
Carbohydrates, 1 serving: 17 g

Yogurt Chocolate Cake

8-oz. pkg.	sugar-free chocolate cake mix	226-g pkg.
1	egg white	1
8 oz.	nonfat plain yogurt	224 g
½ c.	water	125 mL

Combine ingredients in a mixing bowl. Beat on LOW for 1 minute. Continue beating on HIGH 5 minutes more or until batter is thick and very creamy. Transfer to a wax-paper–lined or greased-and-floured 8-in. (20-cm) round cake pan. Bake at 375 °F (190 °C) for 20 to 25 minutes. Cool for 10 minutes in the pan. Turn cake out onto a cooling rack; cool completely.

Yield: 10 servings
Exchange, 1 serving: 1 bread, ½ fat
Calories, 1 serving: 102
Carbohydrates, 1 serving: 18 g

Banana Chocolate Cake

8-oz. pkg.	sugar-free chocolate cake mix	226-g pkg.
1	egg white	1
4-oz. jar	baby banana	113-g jar
⅔ c.	buttermilk	180 mL
⅓ c.	chopped walnuts	90 mL

Combine cake mix, egg white, banana, and buttermilk in a mixing bowl. Beat on LOW for 1 minute. Continue beating on HIGH 5 minutes more or until batter is thick and very creamy. Transfer to a wax-paper–lined or greased-and-floured 8-in. (20-cm) round cake pan. Sprinkle with chopped walnuts. Bake at 375 °F (190 °C) for 20 to 25 minutes. Cool in the pan or serve warm.

Yield: 10 servings
Exchange, 1 serving: 1 bread, 1 fat
Calories, 1 serving: 119
Carbohydrates, 1 serving: 19 g

Yeast Cake

8-oz. pkg.	any sugar-free cake mix	226-g pkg.
1	egg white	1
¼-oz. pkg.	dry yeast	7-g pkg.
⅔ c.	warm water *(not hot)*	180 mL

Combine cake mix, egg white, yeast, and warm water in a mixing bowl. Beat on LOW for 1 minute. Continue beating on HIGH 5 minutes more. Batter will be very thick. Grease and flour a 9-in. (23-cm) round cake pan. Cut a piece of wax paper the size of the bottom of the pan. Fit into the cake pan. Transfer batter to pan. Place a paper towel or wax paper over cake pan. Allow to rise in a warm draft-free area for at least 4 hours. (This cake can rise in the refrigerator in a cake pan covered with wax paper while you are at work during the day or overnight, if you wish to bake it 8 or more hours later.) Bake at 350 °F (175 °C) for 25 to 30 minutes or until tester inserted in middle comes out clean. Cool for 10 minutes in the pan. Turn cake out onto a cooling rack. Remove wax paper. Cool completely or serve warm. This cake is very soft and light.

Yield: 10 servings
Exchange, 1 serving: 1 bread, ½ fat
Calories, 1 serving: 90
Carbohydrates, 1 serving: 16 g

English Pound Cake

8-oz. pkg.	sugar-free pound cake mix	226-g pkg.
1	egg white	1
1 T.	brandy	30 mL
½ t.	ground nutmeg	2 mL
½ t.	ground mace	2 mL
⅔ c.	warm water	180 mL

Combine ingredients in a medium-sized mixing bowl. Beat for 5 minutes. Pour into a wax-paper–lined or greased-and-floured 8 × 4 × 2 in. (20 × 10 × 5 cm) loaf pan, and bake at 350 °F (175 °C) for 45 to 50 minutes. Cool cake in pan for 10 minutes. Turn cake out onto a rack and cool completely or serve warm.

Yield: 10 servings
Exchange, 1 serving: 1 bread, ½ fat
Calories, 1 serving: 90
Carbohydrates, 1 serving: 16 g

Chocolate Pound Cake

1	egg	1
2 oz.	unsweetened chocolate, melted and cooled	57 g
8-oz. pkg.	sugar-free pound cake mix	226-g pkg.
⅔ c.	water	180 mL

Beat egg in a medium-sized mixing bowl until light lemon-colored and fluffy. Beat in cooled chocolate. Add cake mix and water alternately in small amounts, beating well after each addition. Beat a minute more. Pour into a wax-paper–lined or greased-and-floured 8 × 4 × 2 in. (20 × 10 × 5 cm) loaf pan, and bake at 350 °F (175 °C) for 45 to 50 minutes. Cool cake in pan for 10 minutes. Turn cake out onto a rack and cool completely or serve warm.

Yield: 10 servings
Exchange, 1 serving: 1⅓ bread, 1 fat
Calories, 1 serving: 120
Carbohydrates, 1 serving: 20 g

Hazelnut Cake

½ c.	hazelnuts	125 mL
8-oz. pkg.	sugar-free yellow cake mix	226-g pkg.
1	egg white	1
⅔ c.	water	180 mL
1 t.	liquid butter flavoring	5 mL

Place hazelnuts in a food processor or blender. Blend into a fine powder. Combine hazelnut powder, cake mix, and egg white in a mixing bowl. Add water and butter flavoring. Beat on LOW for 1 minute. Continue beating on HIGH 5 minutes more or until batter is thick and very creamy. Transfer to a wax-paper–lined or greased-and-floured 8-in. round cake pan. Bake at 375 °F (190 °C) for 20 to 25 minutes. Cool for 10 minutes in the pan. Turn cake out onto a cooling rack; cool completely.

Yield: 10 servings
Exchange, 1 serving: 1 bread, 1½ fat
Calories, 1 serving: 132
Carbohydrates, 1 serving: 16 g

Pineapple Upside-Down Cake

6	pineapple rings, in juice	6
1 T.	margarine	15 mL
¼ c.	Cary's Sugar-Free Maple-Flavored Syrup	60 mL
1 T.	granulated brown-sugar replacement	15 mL
1 recipe	"Easy Pineapple Cake" (page 38)	1 recipe

Drain juice from pineapple rings. Juice from rings can be used in the preparation of the "Easy Pineapple Cake." Melt margarine in an 8-in. (20-cm) round cake pan. Brush melted margarine over sides and bottom of pan. Cut pineapple rings in half and lay them decoratively on the bottom of the pan. Pour maple syrup over pineapple rings; sprinkle with granulated brown-sugar replacement. Prepare cake as directed in recipe. Pour batter over pineapple rings. Bake at 375 °F (190 °C) for 25 minutes or until tester inserted in middle comes out clean. Immediately turn cake out onto a serving plate. Serve warm. Optional: 1 T. (15 mL) of prepared nondairy whipped topping on each ring to add a pretty and flavorful touch.

Yield: 10 servings
Exchange, 1 serving (without whipped topping): 1 bread, 1 fruit, ½ fat
Calories, 1 serving (without whipped topping): 124
Carbohydrates, 1 serving (without whipped topping): 25 g

Black Cherry Upside-Down Cake

2 T.	margarine	30 mL
2 T.	liquid fructose	30 mL
2 c.	Flavorland frozen dark cherries, thawed	500 mL
2 T.	chopped pecans	30 mL
8-oz. pkg.	Featherlight sugar-free chocolate cake mix	226-g pkg.

Melt margarine in an 8-in. (20-cm) round oven-safe cake pan or skillet. Add liquid fructose and stir until mixed. Add cherries and pecans. Prepare cake mix as directed on package. Pour batter over cherries. Bake at 350 °F (175 °C) for 25 minutes or until tester inserted in middle comes out clean. Turn cake over onto a dessert tray or platter. Serve warm.

Yield: 10 servings
Exchange, 1 serving: 1 bread, ¼ fruit, 1 fat
Calories, 1 serving: 137
Carbohydrates, 1 serving: 20 g

Rhubarb Upside-Down Cake

1 qt.	fresh or frozen rhubarb	1 L
¼ c.	granulated sugar replacement	60 mL
¼ c.	granulated fructose	60 mL
2 T.	cornstarch	30 mL
2 pkgs.	sugar-free yellow cake mix	2 pkgs.
(8-oz.)		(226-g)
1 t.	almond extract	5 mL

Cook rhubarb over low heat until juice begins to run; then add sugar replacement and fructose. Dissolve cornstarch in a small amount of cold water and add to rhubarb mixture. Cook and stir until mixture begins to thicken. Remove from stove. Cool while making cake batter. Combine cake mixes in a large mixing bowl (Remember you have to double the amount of ingredients on the package because you have two cake mixes.) Beat the almond extract into the batter. Pour rhubarb mixture into a greased 8-in.-(20-cm-) square cake pan. Pour batter over rhubarb. Bake at 375 °F (190 °C) for 35 to 45 minutes or until tester inserted in middle comes out clean. Turn out onto a cake plate.

Yield: 16 servings
Exchange, 1 serving: 1¼ bread, ½ fruit, ½ fat
Calories, 1 serving: 122
Carbohydrates, 1 serving: 22 g

Blueberry Jam Cake

1	egg	1
½ c.	all-natural blueberry preserves	125 mL
8-oz. pkg.	sugar-free pound cake mix	226-g pkg.
⅔ c.	water	180 mL

Beat egg in a medium-sized mixing bowl until light lemon-colored and fluffy. Beat in blueberry preserves. Add cake mix and water alternately in small amounts, beating well after each addition. Beat a total of 5 to 6 minutes. Pour into a wax-paper–lined or greased-and-floured 8-in. (20-cm) cake pan, and bake at 350 °F (175 °C) for 20 to 25 minutes. Cool cake in pan for 10 minutes. Turn cake out onto rack and cool completely or serve warm.

Yield: 10 servings
Exchange, 1 serving: 1¼ bread, ½ fruit, ½ fat
Calories, 1 serving: 115
Carbohydrates, 1 serving: 22 g

Lemon Dessert Cake

2 pkgs. (8-oz.)	sugar-free yellow cake mix, prepared	2 pkgs. (226-g)
1 pkg. (4-serving)	lemon-flavored sugar-free instant pudding mix	1 pkg. (4-serving)
1 pkg. (4-serving)	sugar-free lemon gelatin	1 pkg. (4-serving)

Make cakes as directed on package. Then break cakes into medium-size pieces, and lay pieces on the bottom of a 10 × 13 in. (25 × 33 cm) pan. Prepare lemon pudding with skim milk as directed on package. Allow to cool. Prepare lemon gelatin as directed on package. Allow to cool until mixture is softly set. Stir gelatin into pudding. Pour pudding-gelatin mixture over broken cake in pan. Chill thoroughly before serving.

Yield: 20 servings
Exchange, 1 serving: 1 bread, ½ fat
Calories, 1 serving: 96
Carbohydrates, 1 serving: 16 g

Banana Butterscotch Layer Cake

2 pkgs. (8-oz.)	sugar-free yellow cake mix	2 pkgs. (226-g)
1 pkg. (4-serving)	butterscotch-flavored sugar-free instant pudding mix	1 pkg. (4-serving)
2 c.	prepared nondairy whipped topping	500 mL
2	bananas	2

Prepare cake mixes together as directed on package; bake in two 8-in. (20-cm) round pans, with their sides greased and the bottoms lined with wax paper. Allow to cool. Meanwhile, prepare butterscotch pudding as directed on package. Allow to partially set; then stir in nondairy whipped topping. Place one cake upside down on a cake plate or platter. Frost with a thin layer of pudding topping. Cut each banana into very thin slices. Place one of the sliced bananas between the layers. Add the top cake layer, and frost the top and sides of the cake with pudding topping. Decorate top with remaining banana slices.

Yield: 20 servings
Exchange, 1 serving: 1 bread, ¼ fruit, ½ fat
Calories, 1 serving: 118
Carbohydrates, 1 serving: 20 g

Strawberry Dream Cake

2 c.	strawberries, rinsed and hulled	500 mL
1	"Yeast Cake" (page 46), prepared	1
3 c.	prepared nondairy whipped topping	750 mL

Reserve 10 of the best strawberries for garnish. Cut the remaining straw-berries into thick slices. Cut cake in half horizontally. Place bottom half on a serving dessert plate or platter. Cover with 1 c. (250 mL) of the nondairy whipped topping. Place half of the sliced strawberries on top of the whipped topping. Add top layer of cake. Place remaining sliced straw-berries on top of cake. Frost top and sides of cake with remaining whipped topping. Make reserved strawberries into fans by cutting thin lengthwise slices from the tip almost to the stem (do not cut through the stem) and gently fanning out the slices. Place strawberry fans evenly around edge of cake. Chill until serving time.

Yield: 10 servings
Exchange, 1 serving: 1 bread, ½ fat
Calories, 1 serving: 135
Carbohydrates, 1 serving: 23 g

Coconut Cake

1 pkg.	sugar-free white cake mix	1 pkg.
(8-oz.)		(226-g)
¾ c.	unsweetened shredded coconut	190 mL
2 c.	prepared nondairy whipped topping	500 mL

Prepare cake as directed on package, except, after preparing batter, fold in ½ c. (125 mL) of the shredded coconut. Toast remaining ¼ c. (60 mL) of coconut for garnish. (To toast: Place coconut in a small nonstick pan; cook and stir over medium-low heat until coconut is toasted.) Bake cake as directed on package. Allow cake to cool. Frost sides and top of cake with nondairy whipped topping. Sprinkle toasted coconut on top. Refrigerate until ready to serve.

Yield: 10 servings
Exchange, 1 serving: 1 bread, 1 fat
Calories, 1 serving: 147
Carbohydrates, 1 serving: 19 g

Cookies

Cookies conjure up memories of childhood: the sweet smell in the kitchen, a warm cookie melting in your mouth. But many of us just don't have the time to bake those time-consuming delights anymore.

The cookies in this chapter are all made with mixes, so the mixing time is cut to a minimum. I used a hand-held electric mixer or a wooden spoon to mix most of these cookies. Also, there is very little cleanup, the taste is great, and the aroma of these cookies equals that of the most time-consuming recipes.

The best part about cookies is that you can bake many different kinds, freeze them, and eat them when your diet allows it. Cookies—the best dessert ever.

Date Bars

8-oz. pkg.	sugar-free yellow cake mix	226-g pkg.
½ c.	finely chopped dates	125 mL
1	egg white	1
1 T.	low-fat milk	15 mL
24	pecan halves	24

Use a vegetable spray to lightly grease a 7 × 9 in. (17 × 23 cm) baking pan. Combine cake mix and dates in a small bowl. Lightly toss mixture to coat dates with cake mix. Stir in egg white and milk until mixture is well blended. Transfer to greased pan. Press down slightly. Place a pecan half on each section where bar will be cut. Bake at 350 °F (175 °C) for 17 to 20 minutes. Cut and move to cooling rack.

Yield: 24 bars
Exchange, 1 bar: ¾ bread
Calories, 1 bar: 54
Carbohydrates, 1 bar: 9 g

Lemon Almond Cookies

8-oz. pkg.	sugar-free lemon cake mix	226-g pkg.
1 t.	grated lemon peel	5 mL
½ t.	lemon juice	2 mL
½ t.	almond flavoring	2 mL
2 T.	water	30 mL
¼ c.	slivered almonds, toasted	60 mL

Use a vegetable spray to lightly grease the cookie sheets. Combine lemon cake mix, lemon peel, lemon juice, almond flavoring, and water in a small bowl. Use a fork to completely blend. Mix in slivered almonds. Mixture will be large moist crumbs. Lightly dust hands with flour. Form into 30 balls. Place balls on cookie sheets. Bake at 350 °F (175 °C) for 10 to 12 minutes. Allow cookies to cool slightly on sheets before removing.

Yield: 30 cookies
Exchange, 1 cookie: ⅓ bread, ¼ fat
Calories, 1 cookie: 36
Carbohydrates, 1 cookie: 6 g

Chocolate Tubes

12	4-in. (10-cm) wonton wrappers	12
	liquid chocolate flavoring	
1	egg white, slightly beaten	1
1 t.	granulated sugar replacement	5 mL
1½ T.	semisweet chocolate chips	21 mL

Use vegetable spray to lightly grease a cookie sheet. Lay wonton wrappers out on a flat surface. Dip a thin small paintbrush into the chocolate flavoring, and brush four to six stripes down each wrapper. Allow to dry completely. Then turn the wrappers over and brush each one with the beaten egg white. Lightly sprinkle the egg white–brushed side of each wrapper with sugar replacement. Roll each wrapper into a tube with about a ⅜-in. (9-mm) center hole. Place on cookie sheet and bake at 350 °F (175 °C) for 8 to 10 minutes. Remove from sheet and cool completely. Meanwhile, melt the chocolate chips. Dip the ends of each rolled wrapper into the melted chocolate. Allow to cool.

Yield: 12 cookies
Exchange, 1 cookie: negligible
Calories, 1 cookie: negligible
Carbohydrates, 1 cookie: negligible

Raisin Spice Cookies

8-oz. pkg.	sugar-free yellow cake mix	226-g pkg.
3 T.	water	45 mL
1 t.	ground cinnamon	5 mL
¼ t.	ground nutmeg	1 mL
⅛ t.	ground cloves	½ mL
⅓ c.	raisins	90 mL

Use a vegetable spray to lightly grease the cookie sheets. Combine cake mix, water, and spices in a small bowl. Beat thoroughly. Stir in raisins. Drop by teaspoonfuls about 2 in. (5 cm) apart onto the greased cookie sheets. Bake at 350 °F (175 °C) for 10 to 12 minutes.

Yield: 30 cookies
Exchange, 1 cookie: ⅓ bread
Calories, 1 cookie: 33
Carbohydrates, 1 cookie: 7 g

Pistachio Cookies

8-oz. pkg.	sugar-free yellow cake mix	226-g pkg.
¼ c.	finely grated pistachio nuts	60 mL
3 T.	water	45 mL

Use a vegetable spray to lightly grease the cookie sheets. Combine all ingredients in a small bowl. Beat at low speed until mixture is thoroughly blended. Drop by teaspoonfuls about 2 in. (5 cm) apart onto the greased cookie sheets. Bake at 350 °F (175 °C) for 10 to 12 minutes. Allow cookies to cool slightly on sheets before removing.

Yield: 30 cookies
Exchange, 1 cookie: ⅓ bread
Calories, 1 cookie: 28
Carbohydrates, 1 cookie: 4 g

Macaroon Cookies

8-oz. pkg.	sugar-free white cake mix	226-g pkg.
1	egg white	1
1 t.	coconut flavoring	5 mL
2 T.	water	30 mL
¾ c.	unsweetened flaked coconut	190 mL

Use a vegetable spray to lightly grease the cookie sheets. Combine cake mix, egg white, coconut flavoring, and water in a small bowl. Beat at low speed until mixture is thoroughly blended. Blend in the flaked coconut. Drop by teaspoonfuls about 2 in. (5 cm) apart onto the greased cookie sheets. Bake at 375 °F (190 °C) for 9 to 11 minutes. Allow cookies to cool slightly on sheets before removing.

Yield: 40 cookies
Exchange, 1 cookie: ⅓ bread, ¼ fat
Calories, 1 cookie: 35
Carbohydrates, 1 cookie: 4 g

Gingerbread Cookies

8-oz pkg.	sugar-free yellow cake mix	226-g pkg.
½ t.	ground ginger	2 mL
¼ t.	ground nutmeg	1 mL
3 T.	Cary's Sugar-Free Maple-Flavored Syrup	45 mL
2 t.	water	10 mL

Use a vegetable spray to lightly grease the cookie sheets. Combine cake mix, ginger, and nutmeg in a small bowl. Stir to mix. Beat in maple syrup and water. Drop by teaspoonfuls about 2 in. (5 cm) apart onto the greased cookie sheets. Bake at 375 °F (190 °C) for 9 to 11 minutes.

Yield: 30 cookies
Exchange, 1 cookie: ⅓ bread
Calories, 1 cookie: 30
Carbohydrates, 1 cookie: 5 g

Chocolate Chocolate-Chip Cookies

8-oz. pkg.	sugar-free chocolate cake mix	226-g pkg.
3 T.	water	45 mL
¼ c.	semisweet chocolate chips	60 mL

Use a vegetable spray to lightly grease the cookie sheets. Combine cake mix and water in a small bowl. Beat thoroughly. Stir in chocolate chips. Drop by teaspoonfuls about 2 in. (5 cm) apart onto the greased cookie sheets. Bake at 350 °F (175 °C) for 10 to 12 minutes.

Yield: 30 cookies
Exchange, 1 cookie: ⅓ bread, ½ fat
Calories, 1 cookie: 39
Carbohydrates, 1 cookie: 6 g

Anise Cookies

8-oz. pkg.	sugar-free yellow cake mix	226-g pkg.
1 T.	anise seed, crushed	15 mL
3 T.	water	45 mL

Use a vegetable spray to lightly grease the cookie sheets. Combine cake mix, crushed anise seed, and water in a small bowl. Beat thoroughly. Drop by teaspoonfuls about 2 in. (5 cm) apart onto the greased cookie sheets. Bake at 350 °F (175 °C) for 10 to 12 minutes.

Yield: 30 cookies
Exchange, 1 cookie: ⅓ bread
Calories, 1 cookie: 30
Carbohydrates, 1 cookie: 5 g

Fruit Drops

8-oz. pkg.	sugar-free white cake mix	226-g pkg.
3 T.	water	45 mL
⅓ c.	finely chopped mixed dried fruits	90 mL

Use a vegetable spray to lightly grease the cookie sheets. Combine cake mix and water in a small bowl. Beat thoroughly. Fold in chopped fruit. Drop by teaspoonfuls about 2 in. (5 cm) apart onto the greased cookie sheets. Bake at 350 °F (175 °C) for 10 to 12 minutes.

Yield: 30 cookies
Exchange, 1 cookie: ⅓ bread
Calories, 1 cookie: 34
Carbohydrates, 1 cookie: 7 g

Chocolate Cherry Cookies

20	Flavorland frozen tart cherries, thawed with juice	20
8-oz. pkg.	sugar-free chocolate cake mix	226-g pkg.
¼ t.	unsweetened cherry drink mix	1 mL
2 T.	water	30 mL

Use a vegetable spray to lightly grease the cookie sheets. Cut thawed cherries into three or four pieces. Combine chocolate cake mix and cherry drink mix in a small bowl. Add cherries with their juice and the water. Use a fork to thoroughly mix the batter. Batter is quite moist. If you prefer a less soft cookie, use less water. Drop by teaspoonfuls about 2 in. (5 cm) apart ·

onto the greased cookie sheets. Bake at 375 °F (190 °C) for 10 to 12 minutes. Allow cookies to cool slightly on sheets before removing.

Yield: 30 cookies
Exchange, 1 cookie: ⅓ bread
Calories, 1 cookie: 35
Carbohydrates, 1 cookie: 7 g

Chocolate Crunch Cookies

8-oz. pkg.	sugar-free chocolate cake mix	226-g pkg.
¼ t.	lemon flavoring	1 mL
3 T.	water	45 mL
1½ c.	corn flakes	375 mL

Use a vegetable spray to lightly grease the cookie sheets. Combine cake mix, lemon flavoring, and water in a small bowl. Beat to thoroughly blend. Place corn flakes in a bowl. Crush the corn flakes slightly with your hand. Stir into cookie mixture. Drop by teaspoonfuls about 2 in. (5 cm) apart onto the greased cookie sheets. Bake at 375 °F (190 °C) for 10 to 12 minutes. Allow cookies to cool slightly on sheets before removing.

Yield: 40 cookies
Exchange, 1 cookie: ⅓ bread
Calories, 1 cookie: 26
Carbohydrates, 1 cookie: 5 g

Chocolate Coconut Drops

8-oz. pkg.	sugar-free chocolate cake mix	226-g pkg.
¼ t.	lemon flavoring	1 mL
3 T.	water	45 mL
1½ c.	corn flakes	375 mL
½ c.	unsweetened flaked coconut	125 mL

Use a vegetable spray to lightly grease the cookie sheets. Combine all ingredients in a small bowl. Use a fork to thoroughly mix the batter. Cover with plastic wrap and chill for 10 to 15 minutes. Drop by teaspoonfuls about 2 in. (5 cm) apart onto the greased cookie sheets. Bake at 350 °F (175 °C) for 10 to 12 minutes. Allow cookies to cool slightly on sheets before removing.

Yield: 40 cookies
Exchange, 1 cookie: ⅓ bread
Calories, 1 cookie: 30
Carbohydrates, 1 cookie: 5 g

Black-and-White Cookies

8-oz. pkg.	sugar-free chocolate cake mix	226-g pkg.
1	egg white	1
2 T.	water	30 mL
½ c.	white chocolate chips	125 mL

Use a vegetable spray to lightly grease the cookie sheets. Combine chocolate cake mix, egg white, and water in a small bowl. Beat at low speed until mixture is thoroughly blended. Stir in white chocolate chips. Drop by teaspoonfuls about 2 in. (5 cm) apart onto the greased cookie sheets. Bake at 350 °F (175 °C) for 10 to 12 minutes. Allow cookies to cool slightly on sheets before removing.

Yield: 30 cookies
Exchange, 1 cookie: ⅓ bread, ½ fat
Calories, 1 cookie: 44
Carbohydrates, 1 cookie: 6 g

Plain Oatmeal Cookies

8-oz. pkg.	sugar-free white cake mix	226-g pkg.
1	egg white	1
2 T.	water	30 mL
1¼ c.	quick-cooking oatmeal	310 mL

Combine cake mix, egg white, and water in a small bowl. Beat thoroughly. Stir in dry oatmeal. (Add a small amount of extra water, if needed.) Shape into rolls 1½ in. (3.7 cm) in diameter. Wrap in wax paper or plastic wrap. Chill thoroughly. Cut into 40 thin slices. Use a vegetable spray to lightly grease the cookie sheets. Bake at 350 °F (175 °C) for 7 to 9 minutes. Allow cookies to cool slightly on sheets before removing.

Yield: 40 cookies
Exchange, 1 cookie: ⅓ bread
Calories, 1 cookie: 32
Carbohydrates, 1 cookie: 5 g

Chocolate Oatmeal Rounds

8-oz. pkg.	sugar-free chocolate cake mix	226-g pkg.
1	egg white	1
2 T.	water	30 mL
1¼ c.	quick-cooking oatmeal	310 mL

Combine chocolate cake mix, egg white, and water in a small bowl. Beat thoroughly. Stir in dry oatmeal. Add a small amount of water, if needed. Shape into rolls 1½ in. (3.7 cm) in diameter. Wrap in wax paper or plastic wrap. Chill thoroughly. Cut into 40 thin slices. Use a vegetable spray to lightly grease the cookie sheets. Bake at 350 °F (175 °C) for 7 to 9 minutes. Allow cookies to cool slightly on sheet before removing.

Yield: 40 cookies
Exchange, 1 cookie: ½ bread
Calories, 1 cookie: 35
Carbohydrates, 1 cookie: 7 g

Chocolate Sour-Cream Cookies

8-oz. pkg.	sugar-free chocolate cake mix	226-g pkg.
3 T.	sour cream	45 mL
1 t.	water	5 mL

Use a vegetable spray to lightly grease the cookie sheets. Combine cake mix, sour cream, and water in a small bowl. Beat thoroughly. Drop from a teaspoon onto the greased cookie sheets. Bake at 350 °F (175 °C) for 9 to 10 minutes.

Yield: 30 cookies
Exchange, 1 cookie: ⅓ bread
Calories, 1 cookie: 33
Carbohydrates, 1 cookie: 5 g

Apple Cookies

| 1 | Granny Smith apple, peeled and chopped | 1 |
| 8-oz. pkg. | sugar-free white cake mix | 226-g pkg. |

Use a vegetable spray to lightly grease the cookie sheets. Place apple in a micro-safe bowl. Cover and cook on HIGH for 2 minutes, stirring after 1 minute. Uncover and continue cooking on MEDIUM until apple mixture is very thick and tender. Cool. Stir in cake mix. Drop from a teaspoon about 2 in. (5 cm) apart onto the greased cookie sheets. Bake at 375 °F (190 °C) for 8 to 10 minutes.

Yield: 30 cookies
Exchange, 1 cookie: ⅓ bread
Calories, 1 cookie: 36
Carbohydrates, 1 cookie: 6 g

Brandy Lizzies

8-oz. pkg.	sugar-free yellow cake mix	226-g pkg.
1	egg white	1
2 T.	water	30 mL
1 t.	brandy flavoring	5 mL
1 c.	quick-cooking oatmeal	250 mL
½ c.	raisins, chopped	125 mL
¼ c.	pecans, chopped	60 mL

Combine cake mix, egg white, water, and brandy flavoring in a small bowl. Beat thoroughly. Stir in dry oatmeal, raisins, and pecans. Chill for 2 hours. Use a vegetable spray to lightly grease the cookie sheets. Drop from a teaspoon onto the greased cookie sheets. Bake at 350 °F (175 °C) for 9 to 10 minutes.

Yield: 40 cookies
Exchange, 1 cookie: ⅓ bread, ¼ fat
Calories, 1 cookie: 36
Carbohydrates, 1 cookie: 6 g

Tart Lemon Cookies

2 T.	low-fat milk	30 mL
2 t.	white vinegar	10 mL
8-oz. pkg.	sugar-free lemon cake mix	226-g pkg.
½ t.	grated lemon peel	2 mL

Use a vegetable spray to lightly grease the cookie sheets. Combine milk and vinegar in a small bowl. Stir to blend. Stir in lemon cake mix and lemon peel. Drop from a teaspoon about 2 in. (5 cm) apart onto the greased cookie sheets. Bake at 350 °F (175 °C) for 9 to 10 minutes. Carefully remove from pan immediately.

Yield: 30 cookies
Exchange, 1 cookie: ⅓ bread
Calories, 1 cookie: 35
Carbohydrates, 1 cookie: 6 g

Great Pumpkin Cookies

8-oz. pkg.	sugar-free carrot cake mix	226-g pkg.
3 T.	pumpkin puree	45 mL
	nutmeg	

Use a vegetable spray to grease the cookie sheets. Combine carrot cake mix and pumpkin puree in a small bowl. Beat to blend. Drop from a teaspoon about 2 in. (5 cm) apart onto the greased cookie sheets. Sprinkle with a little nutmeg. Bake at 350 °F (175 °C) for 8 to 9 minutes.

Yield: 30 cookies
Exchange, 1 cookie: ⅓ bread
Calories, 1 cookie: 33
Carbohydrates, 1 cookie: 5 g

Maple Mellow Bars

Base

8-oz. pkg.	sugar-free pound cake mix	226-g pkg.
1	egg white	1

Topping

2	egg whites	2
¼ t.	maple flavoring	1 mL
dash	salt	dash
¼ t.	cream of tartar	1 mL
¼ t.	ground cinnamon	1 mL
¼ t.	ground nutmeg	1 mL
dash	ground ginger	dash

Use vegetable spray to grease an 8-in.- (20-cm-) square baking pan. Combine pound cake mix and the one egg white in a small bowl. Use a fork to blend ingredients together thoroughly. Set aside ⅓ cup (90 mL) of the cake mixture. Press remaining cake mixture into the bottom of the greased pan. Combine the two egg whites, maple flavoring, and salt in a mixing bowl. Beat into soft peaks. Add cream of tartar and continue beating until stiff. Spread onto pressed-cake mixture in the pan. To the reserved ⅓ c. (90 mL) of cake mixture, add cinnamon, nutmeg, and ginger. Work with a fork until spices are completely incorporated into the cake mixture. Sprinkle spiced mixture on top of beaten egg whites in pan. Bake at 350 °F (175 °C) for 20 minutes. Cut into 24 bars. Remove from pan and cool on rack.

Yield: 24 bars
Exchange, 1 bar: ⅓ bread, ½ fat
Calories, 1 bar: 44
Carbohydrates, 1 bar: 5 g

Peanut Butter Mellow Bars

Base

8-oz. pkg.	sugar-free white cake mix	226-g pkg.
¼ c.	chunky peanut butter	60 mL
2 t.	water	10 mL

Topping

2	egg whites	2
¼ t.	vanilla flavoring	1 mL
dash	salt	dash
¼ t.	cream of tartar	1 mL
2 T.	finely ground salted peanuts	30 mL

Use vegetable spray to grease an 8-in.- (20-cm-) square baking pan. Combine white cake mix and peanut butter in a small bowl. Use a fork to thoroughly blend. Set aside ¼ c. (60 mL) of the cake mixture. Add the 2 t. (10 mL) of water to remaining cake mixture and blend. Press cake mixture into the bottom of the greased pan. Combine the two egg whites, vanilla flavoring, and salt in a mixing bowl. Beat into soft peaks. Add cream of tartar and continue beating until stiff. Spread onto pressed-cake mixture in the pan. To the reserved ¼ c. (60 mL) of cake mixture, add ground salted peanuts. Stir to mix. Sprinkle mixture on top of beaten egg whites in pan. Bake at 350 °F (175 °C) for 20 minutes. Cut into 24 bars. Remove from pan and cool on rack.

Yield: 24 bars
Exchange, 1 bar: ½ bread, ½ fat
Calories, 1 bar: 53
Carbohydrates, 1 bar: 7 g

Frosted Ginger Creams

8-oz. pkg.	sugar-free carrot cake mix	226-g pkg.
1	egg, slightly beaten	1
½ t.	burnt sugar flavoring	2 mL
½ t.	ground ginger	2 mL
1 T.	sugar-free vanilla frosting mix	15 mL
2½ t.	water	12 mL

Use a vegetable spray to grease well an 8-in.- (20-cm-) square baking pan. Combine carrot cake mix, egg, burnt sugar flavoring, and ginger in a small bowl. Beat to blend. Transfer to greased baking pan. Bake at 350 °F (175 °C) for 17 to 20 minutes. Cool in pan. Combine vanilla frosting mix and water in a small cup. Stir with a fork to thoroughly mix. Drizzle over cookies. Cut into 24 bars.

Yield: 24 bars
Exchange, 1 bar: ½ bread
Calories, 1 bar: 43
Carbohydrates, 1 bar: 7 g

Peanut Chocolate Bars

Use "Peanut Butter Mellow Bars" recipe on opposite page. Before spreading stiffly beaten egg whites on base, sprinkle base with ¼ c. (60 mL) of semisweet chocolate chips that have been chopped into fine pieces. Or melt the chips and spread with the melted chocolate. Proceed with recipe.

Yield: 24 bars
Exchange, 1 bar: ½ bread, ½ fat
Calories, 1 bar: 62
Carbohydrates, 1 bar: 8 g

Walnut Brownies

8-oz. pkg.	sugar-free chocolate cake mix	226-g pkg.
1	egg yolk, beaten	1
1 T.	water	5 mL
¼ t.	vanilla flavoring	1 mL
⅓ c.	chopped walnuts	90 mL

Use a vegetable spray to lightly grease an 8-in.- (20-cm-) square cake pan. Combine chocolate cake mix, egg yolk, water, and vanilla flavoring in a small bowl. Stir to completely blend. Transfer mixture to greased pan. Sprinkle with walnuts. Bake at 350 °F (175 °C) for 17 to 20 minutes. Cut and move from pan to cooling rack.

Yield: 24 bars
Exchange, 1 bar: ⅓ bread, ½ fat
Calories, 1 bar: 48
Carbohydrates, 1 bar: 5 g

Coconut Dream Squares

Base

1 c.	quick-cooking oatmeal	250 mL
3 T.	granulated brown-sugar replacement	45 mL
1	egg, slightly beaten	1

Topping

2	eggs	2
3 T.	granulated brown-sugar replacement	45 mL
1 t.	vanilla flavoring	5 mL
1 c.	unsweetened shredded coconut	250 mL
½ t.	baking powder	2 mL

Use vegetable spray to grease an 8-in.- (20-cm-) square baking pan. Combine dry oatmeal, 3 T. (45 mL) of the brown-sugar replacement, and the one egg in a small bowl. Stir to blend thoroughly. Transfer to greased pan. Flour hands and press into bottom of pan. Bake at 350 °F (175 °C) for 6 to 7 minutes or until base is set. Combine the two eggs and 3 T. (45 mL) of the brown-sugar replacement for topping in a bowl. Beat with a fork. Stir in vanilla flavoring, shredded coconut, and baking powder. Pour mixture over warm base. Spread evenly. Continue baking at 350 °F (175 °C) 20 to 22 minutes more or until top is lightly browned and mixture is set. Cut into 36 squares.

Yield: 36 squares
Exchange, 1 square: ½ fat
Calories, 1 square: 20
Carbohydrates, 1 square: 2 g

Butterscotch Bars

2	eggs	2
½ c.	granulated brown-sugar replacement	125 mL
1 t.	butterscotch flavoring	5 mL
8-oz. pkg.	sugar-free yellow cake mix	226-g pkg.
¼ c.	chopped walnuts	60 mL

Use a vegetable spray to slightly grease a 7 × 11 in. (17 × 27 cm) baking pan. Beat eggs; then stir in brown-sugar replacement. Add remaining ingredients and blend thoroughly. Transfer to greased baking pan. Bake at 350 °F (175 °C) for 15 to 17 minutes. Cut into 30 bars, and move from pan to cooling rack.

Yield: 30 bars
Exchange, 1 bar: ⅓ bread, ½ fat
Calories, 1 bar: 42
Carbohydrates, 1 bar: 6 g

Chocolate Pecan Sticks

8-oz. pkg.	sugar-free chocolate cake mix	226-g pkg.
⅓ c.	quick-cooking oatmeal	90 mL
2	egg whites	2
1 t.	vanilla flavoring	5 mL
⅓ c.	chopped pecans	90 mL

Use a vegetable spray to lightly grease a 7 × 11 in. (17 × 27 cm) baking pan. Combine chocolate cake mix, dry oatmeal, one of the egg whites, and vanilla flavoring in a small bowl. Use a fork to thoroughly blend. Press mixture into bottom of greased pan. Beat remaining egg white slightly and brush over top of dough. Sprinkle evenly with chopped pecans. Bake at 350 °F (175 °C) for 15 to 17 minutes. Cut into 30 sticks, and move from pan to cooling rack.

Yield: 30 sticks
Exchange, 1 stick: ⅓ bread, ¼ fat
Calories, 1 stick: 41
Carbohydrates, 1 stick: 6 g

Mocha Fruit Nut Drops

1 T.	instant coffee powder	15 mL
3 T.	water	45 mL
8-oz. pkg.	sugar-free chocolate cake mix	226-g pkg.
¼ c.	coarsely chopped black walnuts	60 mL
¼ c.	chopped dates	60 mL

Use a vegetable spray to lightly grease the cookie sheets. Dissolve the coffee powder in the water. Combine the coffee water and chocolate cake mix in a small mixing bowl. Beat to blend. Fold in nuts and dates. Drop from a teaspoon about 2 in. (5 cm) apart onto the greased cookie sheets. Bake at 350 °F (175 °C) for 9 to 10 minutes.

Yield: 36 cookies
Exchange, 1 cookie: ⅓ bread
Calories, 1 cookie: 34
Carbohydrates, 1 cookie: 6 g

Peanut Sticks

2 c.	quick-cooking oatmeal	500 mL
½ c.	finely ground salted peanuts	125 mL
1 T.	granulated fructose	15 mL
1 t.	baking powder	5 mL
¼ c.	peanut butter	60 mL
2	eggs	2

Use a vegetable spray to lightly grease a 7 × 11 in. (17 × 27 cm) baking pan. Combine dry oatmeal, ground peanuts, fructose, and baking powder in a small bowl. Mix slightly. Beat peanut butter and eggs together thoroughly. Stir into dry mixture until thoroughly mixed. Transfer mixture to greased baking pan. Use the back of a spoon to press mixture evenly into the bottom of the pan. Bake at 350 °F (175 °C) for 15 minutes. Remove from oven. Cut into 27 sticks, and transfer to cooling rack.

Yield: 27 sticks
Exchange, 1 stick: ⅓ bread, ½ fat
Calories, 1 bar: 53
Carbohydrates, 1 bar: 5 g

Frosted Oatmeal Bars

2 c.	quick-cooking oatmeal	500 mL
3 T.	granulated fructose	45 mL
1 t.	baking powder	5 mL
2	eggs, slightly beaten	2
¼ c.	mini–chocolate chips	60 mL

Use a vegetable spray to lightly grease a 7 × 11 in. (17 × 27 cm) baking pan. Combine dry oatmeal, fructose, and baking powder in a small bowl. Mix slightly. Stir in eggs until thoroughly mixed. Transfer mixture to greased baking pan. Use the back of a spoon to press mixture evenly into the bottom of the pan. Bake at 350 °F (175 °C) for 15 minutes. Remove from oven. Sprinkle mini–chocolate chips evenly over surface. Return to oven and bake 2 to 3 minutes more or until chips are very soft. Spread melted chips around top. Cut into 30 bars, and transfer to cooling rack.

Yield: 30 bars
Exchange, 1 bar: ⅓ bread
Calories, 1 bar: 49
Carbohydrates, 1 bar: 5 g

Lunch Box Raisin Bran Bars

2	egg whites	2
dash	salt and nutmeg	dash
½ t.	vanilla flavoring	2 mL
½ t.	cream of tartar	2 mL
3 c.	raisin bran cereal	750 mL

Line an 8-in.- (20-cm-) square pan with wax paper. Combine egg whites, salt, nutmeg, and vanilla flavoring in a small bowl. Beat to soft peaks; then add cream of tartar. Continue beating to firm peaks. Fold in raisin bran cereal thoroughly. Pack mixture into wax-paper–lined pan. Bake at 350 °F (175 °C) for 15 minutes. Remove pan from oven. Cut around edge of pan to loosen any part that is stuck to the side. Turn out onto a cutting board. Carefully remove wax paper. Cut into 20 bars with a scissors.

Yield: 20 bars
Exchange, 1 bar: ⅓ bread
Calories, 1 bar: 29
Carbohydrates, 1 bar: 4 g

Ribbon Cookies

12	4-in. (10-cm) wonton wrappers	12
1	egg white, slightly beaten	1
1 t.	granulated sugar replacement	5 mL
1 T.	sugar-free white frosting mix	15 mL
	water	
2 T.	multicolored cereal balls, crushed fine	30 mL

Use vegetable spray to lightly grease a cookie sheet. Brush each wonton wrapper with the beaten egg white. Lightly sprinkle the egg white–brushed side of each wrapper with sugar replacement. Roll each wrapper into a tube with about a ⅜-in. (9-mm) center hole. Place on cookie sheet and bake at 350 °F (175 °C) for 8 to 10 minutes. Remove from sheet and cool completely. Meanwhile, mix the frosting mix with a small amount of water to make a glaze. Using a small paintbrush, coat the top of each cooled wrapper. Lay wrappers on wax paper. Sprinkle with crushed multicolored cereal balls.

Yield: 12 cookies
Exchange, 1 cookie: negligible
Calories, 1 cookie: negligible
Carbohydrates, 1 cookie: negligible

Sweet Cinnamon Flats

12	4-in. (10-cm) wonton wrappers	12
1	egg white, slightly beaten	1
1 T.	granulated sugar replacement	15 mL
1 t.	ground cinnamon	5 mL

Use vegetable spray to lightly grease a cookie sheet. Brush each won-ton wrapper with the beaten egg white. Lightly sprinkle the egg white–brushed side of each wrapper with sugar replacement and cinnamon. Lay flat on the cookie sheet and bake at 350 °F (175 °C) for 8 to 10 minutes. Remove from sheet and cool completely.

Yield: 12 cookies
Exchange, 1 cookie: negligible
Calories, 1 cookie: negligible
Carbohydrates, 1 cookie: negligible

Lemon Dainties

| 1 | large egg | 1 |
| 8-oz. pkg. | sugar-free lemon cake mix | 226-g pkg. |

Beat large egg until light and fluffy. Beat in half of the lemon cake mix until creamy. Thoroughly stir in remaining cake mix with a fork. Drop from a teaspoon about 2 in. (5 cm) apart onto ungreased cookie sheets. Bake at 350 °F (175 °C) for 9 to 10 minutes or until edges of cookies are delicately tanned. Carefully remove from pan immediately.

Yield: 30 cookies
Exchange, 1 cookie: ⅓ bread
Calories, 1 cookie: 33
Carbohydrates, 1 cookie: 5 g

Strawberry Cream Cookies

2 T.	strawberry-flavored cream cheese	30 mL
3 T.	Cary's Sugar-Free Maple-Flavored Syrup	45 mL
8-oz. pkg.	sugar-free yellow cake mix	226-g pkg.
4 t.	all-natural fruit preserves	20 mL

Use a vegetable spray to lightly grease the cookie sheets. Combine cream cheese and maple syrup in a small bowl. Cream thoroughly. Beat in cake mix until mixture is moist and in large crumbs. Chill at least 10 minutes.

Lightly dust hands with flour. Form dough into 30 balls. Place balls on cookie sheets about 2 in. (5 cm) apart. Press center of each with thumb. Bake at 350 °F (175 °C) for 5 minutes. Remove from oven and press down centers again. Continue baking 5 to 6 minutes more. Cool slightly and fill centers with preserves.

Yield: 30 cookies
Exchange, 1 cookie: ⅓ bread
Calories, 1 cookie: 33
Carbohydrates, 1 cookie: 6 g

Peanut Butter Balls

⅓ c.	peanut butter	90 mL
8-oz. pkg.	sugar-free white cake mix	226-g pkg.
2 T.	water	30 mL

Use a vegetable spray to lightly grease the cookie sheets. Cream peanut butter in a small bowl. Add cake mix and water. Beat at low speed until mixture is thoroughly blended. Mixture will be large moist crumbs. Form into 30 balls. Place balls on cookie sheet. Bake at 350 °F (175 °C) for 10 to 12 minutes. Allow cookies to cool slightly on sheets before removing.

Yield: 30 cookies
Exchange, 1 cookie: ⅓ bread, ½ fat
Calories, 1 cookie: 49
Carbohydrates, 1 cookie: 6 g

Pies

Pies have always been a favorite dessert with family and friends. But never before have pies been so easy to make. Today food manufacturers have taken both the time and the guesswork out of making a good pastry shell, by producing ready-to-bake preformed shells, flat pie sheets that are already cut to an 8- or 9-in. (20- or 23-cm)-size pan, pie sticks that you crumb and then add a small amount of water to and roll yourself, and pie crumbs of all kinds. In addition, there are recipes that you can use to make your own pastry shells. So, there are many options for you to choose from.

In this book, I have basically made all one-crust pies, thus eliminating the extra calories and exchanges of a second crust. To make pies even faster, you can prebake your single shell and freeze it until you need it. All of the nutritional values are given for only the filling, unless otherwise stated. Therefore, if you wish, you can make just the pie filling and place it in individual-serving dishes without any crust or with a pastry-cutout decoration or crumb topping. If you use a shell or topping, remember to add the exchanges, calories, and carbohydrates to those of your pie filling.

Products from Food Manufacturers

Preformed pie shells, for 8-in. (20-cm) pie or tart pans:

Frozen Plain Flour Shells
Yield: 8 servings
Exchange, 1 serving: 1 bread, 1 fat
Calories, 1 serving: 110
Carbohydrates, 1 serving: 14 g

Plain Graham Cracker Shells
Yield: 8 servings
Exchange, 1 serving: 1 bread, 1 fat
Calories, 1 serving: 110
Carbohydrates, 1 serving: 14 g

Chocolate-Flavored Shells
Yield: 8 servings
Exchange, 1 serving: 1 bread, 1 fat
Calories, 1 serving: 120
Carbohydrates, 1 serving: 16 g

Pie sheets, for 8- or 9-in. (20- or 23-cm) pie or tart pans, found in refrigerator section of supermarket:

Yield: 8 servings
Exchange, 1 serving: 1 bread, 1 fat
Calories, 1 serving: 120
Carbohydrates, 1 serving: 12 g

Pie cracker crumbs and flour mixes, for 8- or 9-in. (20- or 23-cm) pie or tart pans, found on supermarket shelf:

Yield: 8 servings
Exchange, 1 serving: 1 bread, 1 fat
Calories, 1 serving: 120
Carbohydrates, 1 serving: 12 g

Pastry for Single-Crust Pie

¼ c.	cold vegetable shortening	60 mL
¾ c.	all-purpose flour	190 mL
dash	salt	dash
2 T.	cold water	30 mL

Place shortening, flour, and salt in an electric mixing bowl or food processor. Beat at low speed until mixture is consistency of coarse oatmeal. Add cold water all at one time, and continue mixing on LOW for 15 to 20 seconds or until mixture clings together. Shape dough into a ball. Dough should feel moist. On lightly floured surface, roll pastry into about a 10-in. (25-cm) circle. Fold rolled dough in half or quarters, and gently fit into pie or tart pan. Gently press dough to sides of pan. Fold under or cut off edge of crust. Decorate edge as desired. Prick entire surface evenly and closely with a fork. If time allows, chill dough thoroughly, at least ½ hour. Bake at 450 °F (230 °C) for 10 to 15 minutes or until nicely browned. Cool before filling.

Yield: 8 servings
Exchange, 1 serving: ½ bread, 1 fat
Calories, 1 serving: 95
Carbohydrates, 1 serving: 8 g

Crumb Pie Shells

1¼ c.	fine crumbs (graham cracker, dry cereal, zwieback)	310 mL
3 T.	melted margarine	45 mL
1 T.	water	15 mL
	spices, flavoring, or sugar replacement (optional)*	

*If using a liquid flavoring or sugar replacement, it must be part of the measured water amount.

Combine crumbs with melted margarine and water; add optional ingredients, if desired. Blend until crumbly. Press crumbs evenly on bottom and sides of 8- or 9-in. (20- or 23-cm) pie or tart pan. Either chill until set or bake at 325 °F (165 °C) for 8 to 10 minutes. Cool before filling.

Yield: 8 servings
Exchange, 1 serving: ⅓ bread, 1 fat
Calories, 1 serving: 67
Carbohydrates, 1 serving: 4 g

Pastry Cutouts and Lattice Tops

Use the extra dough cut from any flour pie shell or make extra dough. Roll the dough as you would for the shell.

For cutouts: Cut with a cookie cutter, in diamonds, hearts, leaves, dots, or strips. Place on cookie sheet.

For lattice or strip top: On a cookie sheet, weave crosswise strips of pastry under and over lengthwise strips of pastry, and cut around edge to form a circle about the size of the top of your pie.

Prick with a fork, and bake at 425 °F (220 °C) for 6 to 8 minutes or until golden brown.

Nutritional value, 2-in. square per serving: negligible

Sweet Streusel Topping

½ c.	all-purpose flour	125 mL
¼ c.	cold margarine	60 mL
3 T.	granulated fructose	45 mL

Combine ingredients in a bowl. Cut through mixture until completely mixed. Sprinkle on top of pie filling. (If desired, place under broiler for 1 or 2 minutes until lightly browned.)

Yield: 8 servings
Exchange, 1 serving: ½ bread, 1 fat
Calories, 1 serving: 90
Carbohydrates, 1 serving: 7 g

Spicy Pecan Topping

¼ c.	cold margarine	60 mL
¼ c.	brown-sugar replacement	60 mL
⅓ c.	all-purpose flour	90 mL
½ t.	ground cinnamon	2 mL
¼ c.	chopped pecans	60 mL

Combine margarine, brown-sugar replacement, flour, and cinnamon in a bowl. Mix until completely blended. Stir in pecans. Sprinkle on top of pie filling. (If desired, place under oven broiler for 1 or 2 minutes until lightly browned.)

Yield: 8 servings
Exchange, 1 serving: ¼ bread, 1 fat
Calories, 1 serving: 73
Carbohydrates, 1 serving: 4 g

Sugar-Replacement Oatmeal Topping

½ c.	quick-cooking oatmeal	125 mL
¼ c.	all-purpose flour	60 mL
¼ c.	brown-sugar replacement	60 mL
¼ c.	cold margarine	60 mL

Combine ingredients in a bowl. Cut through mixture until completely mixed. Sprinkle on top of pie filling. (If desired, place under broiler for 1 to 2 minutes or until lightly browned.)

Yield: 8 servings
Exchange, 1 serving: ⅓ bread, 1 fat
Calories, 1 serving: 83
Carbohydrates, 1 serving: 6 g

Toasted Oatmeal Topping

¼ c.	margarine	60 mL
1 c.	quick-cooking oatmeal	250 mL
2 T.	granulated fructose	30 mL

Melt margarine in a skillet. Stir in oatmeal and fructose. Cook and stir until oatmeal is toasted. Sprinkle on top of pie filling. (If desired, place under broiler for 1 to 2 minutes until lightly browned.)

Yield: 8 servings
Exchange, 1 serving: ½ bread, 1½ fat
Calories, 1 serving: 97
Carbohydrates, 1 serving: 9 g

Cinnamon Pecan Topping

¼ c.	chopped pecans	60 mL
1 t.	granulated fructose	5 mL
¼ t.	ground cinnamon	1 mL

Mix together. Sprinkle over cooled pie filling.

Yield: 8 servings
Exchange, 1 serving: ¾ fat
Calories, 1 serving: 27
Carbohydrates, 1 serving: negligible

Toasted Coconut Topping

¼ c.	grated or shredded unsweetened coconut	60 mL

Place coconut in a small skillet. Toast over medium heat on top of stove, stirring constantly. Sprinkle on top of pie filling.

Yield: 8 servings
Exchange, 1 serving: ⅓ fat
Calories, 1 serving: 17
Carbohydrates, 1 serving: negligible

Favorite Blueberry Pie

	baked pastry shell	
2 bags	Flavorland frozen blueberries	2 bags
(16-oz.)		(453-g)
1 c.	cold water	250 mL
⅓ c.	all-purpose flour	90 mL
¼ c.	granulated fructose	60 mL
1 t.	grated lemon peel	5 mL

Remove 1 c. (250 mL) of blueberries from one of the bags. Set aside reserved blueberries and allow the rest to partially thaw. Combine cold water, flour, and fructose in a saucepan. Stir to dissolve flour. Cook and stir over medium heat until mixture is a very thick paste. Fold partially frozen blueberries into paste mixture until all berries are coated and mixture is evenly distributed throughout the berries. Stir in grated lemon peel. Transfer to bottom of baked pastry shell. Arrange evenly. Top with reserved blueberries. Chill thoroughly.

Yield: 8 servings
Exchange, 1 serving (without pastry shell): 1½ fruit
Calories, 1 serving (without pastry shell): 90
Carbohydrates, 1 serving (without pastry shell): 21 g

Cranberry Blueberry Pie

	baked pastry shell	
2 c.	fresh cranberries, grated	500 mL
1 c.	water	250 mL
3 T.	cornstarch	45 mL
½ c.	granulated fructose	125 mL
2 c.	frozen blueberries, partially thawed	500 mL

Combine cranberries, water, cornstarch, and fructose in a saucepan. Cook and stir over medium heat until mixture is very thick. Fold partially frozen blueberries into mixture until all berries are coated and mixture is evenly distributed throughout the berries. Transfer to bottom of baked pastry shell. Arrange evenly. If desired, decorate top with pastry cutouts. Chill thoroughly.

Yield: 8 servings
Exchange, 1 serving (without pastry shell): 1 fruit
Calories, 1 serving (without pastry shell): 49
Carbohydrates, 1 serving (without pastry shell): 11 g

Black Bottom Lemon Cream Pie

	baked pastry shell	
2 pkgs. (4-serving)	sugar-free lemon gelatin	2 pkgs. (4-serving)
2 t.	grated lemon rind	10 mL
½ c.	sugarless carob drops	125 mL
1 c.	prepared nondairy whipped topping	250 mL

In a large bowl, prepare lemon gelatin as directed on package with the addition of the lemon rind. Set completely. Melt carob drops over hot water. Spread evenly over bottom of pastry shell. With an electric mixer, beat the set gelatin until fluffy. Beat in the nondairy whipped topping. Pile gelatin mixture into pastry shell. Chill thoroughly.

Yield: 8 servings
Exchange, 1 serving (without pastry shell): ½ bread
Calories, 1 serving (without pastry shell): 48
Carbohydrates, 1 serving (without pastry shell): 8 g

Black Raspberry and Strawberry Layered Pie

baked pastry shell

For strawberry layer:

16-oz. bag	Flavorland frozen strawberries	453-g bag
⅔ c.	water	180 mL
2 T.	cornstarch	30 mL
2 T.	granulated fructose	30 mL
1 t.	strawberry flavoring	5 mL

For black raspberry layer:

12-oz. bag	Flavorland frozen black raspberries	340-g bag
½ c.	water	125 mL
2 T.	cornstarch	30 mL
2 T.	granulated fructose	30 mL
1 t.	vanilla flavoring or extract	5 mL
½ t.	grated orange peel	2 mL

For strawberry layer:

Remove four large frozen strawberries from bag. Set aside reserved strawberries and allow remaining strawberries to partially thaw. Combine water, cornstarch, fructose, and strawberry flavoring in a saucepan. Cook and stir over medium heat until mixture is a very thick paste. Mixture will not be clear. Fold partially frozen strawberries into paste mixture until all berries are coated and mixture is clear. (If not clear, return to stove and heat slightly. Cool completely.) Set aside.

For black raspberry layer:

Partially thaw black raspberries. Combine water, cornstarch, fructose, vanilla, and orange peel in a saucepan. Cook and stir over medium heat until mixture is a very thick paste. Fold partially frozen black raspberries into paste mixture until all berries are coated and mixture is clear. (If not clear, return to stove and heat slightly. Cool completely before continuing.)

To complete pie:

Transfer strawberry mixture to bottom of baked pastry shell. Arrange evenly. Top with black raspberry mixture. Cut the four reserved strawberries in half lengthwise, and decorate with the eight halves around the top of the pie. Chill thoroughly.

Yield: 8 servings
Exchange, 1 serving (without pastry shell): 1¼ fruit
Calories, 1 serving (without pastry shell): 72
Carbohydrates, 1 serving (without pastry shell): 18 g

Mocha Pie

	pastry shell, baked	
2 pkgs.	chocolate-flavored sugar-free	2 pkgs.
(4-serving)	to-cook pudding mix	(4-serving)
3 c.	skim milk	750 mL
1 c.	cold strong coffee	250 mL
2 c.	prepared nondairy whipped topping	500 mL

Combine chocolate pudding mix, milk, and coffee in a saucepan. Cook and stir over medium heat until mixture comes to a full boil. Allow to cool for 5 to 10 minutes. Transfer to pastry shell. Refrigerate until completely set. Decorate with the nondairy whipped topping before serving.

Yield: 8 servings
Exchange, 1 serving (without pastry shell): 1 skim milk, ½ fat
Calories, 1 serving (without pastry shell): 109
Carbohydrates, 1 serving (without pastry shell): 14 g

Rhubarb Pie

	baked pastry shell	
2 pkgs.	frozen rhubarb, thawed	2 pkgs.
(1-lb.)		(453-g)
½ c.	granulated fructose	125 mL
¼ c.	water	60 mL
3 T.	all-purpose flour	45 mL
1 t.	vanilla flavoring or extract	5 mL

Place rhubarb and fructose in a saucepan or microwave bowl. Cook over medium heat until rhubarb is almost tender. Combine water and flour in a shaker bottle or small bowl. Shake or beat to completely blend. Pour into rhubarb mixture. Cook and stir until mixture is very thick and rhubarb is tender. Remove from heat. Stir in vanilla. Cool slightly. Transfer to baked pastry shell. Refrigerate thoroughly.

Yield: 8 servings
Exchange, 1 serving (without pastry shell): ¾ fruit
Calories, 1 serving (without pastry shell): 47
Carbohydrates, 1 serving (without pastry shell): 11 g

Old-Fashioned Lemon Meringue Pie

	baked pastry shell	
¾ c.	granulated fructose	190 mL
1 c.	water	250 mL
¼ t.	salt	1 mL
½ c.	cornstarch	125 mL
¾ c.	water	190 mL
4	egg yolks, slightly beaten	4
½ c.	lemon juice	125 mL
2 T.	margarine	30 mL
2 t.	grated lemon rind	10 mL
4	egg whites	4
¼ t.	cream of tartar	1 mL
2 T.	granulated fructose	30 mL
2 T.	granulated sugar replacement	30 mL

Combine the ¾ c. (190 mL) of fructose, the 1 c. (250 mL) of water, and salt in a saucepan. Stir and cook until boiling. Combine cornstarch and the ¾ c. (190 mL) of water in a shaker bottle or small bowl, and mix thoroughly. Stir cornstarch mixture slowly into boiling fructose mixture. Cook until thick and clear. Remove from heat. Combine beaten egg yolks and lemon juice. Stir into thickened hot mixture. Return to heat and continue cooking, stirring constantly until mixture boils rapidly again. Remove from heat; then stir in margarine and lemon rind. Cover and cool to lukewarm. Transfer to baked pastry shell.

For meringue: Combine egg whites and cream of tartar in a mixing bowl, and beat until frothy. Combine the 2 T. (30 mL) of fructose and the sugar replacement in a small cup. Continue beating egg whites, gradually adding combined sweeteners, until stiff.

Pile meringue on top of lemon filling in pastry shell. Spread evenly over filling, including crust of shell. Bake at 325 °F (165 °C) for about 5 minutes or until lightly browned. Move pie to rack and cool completely.

Yield: 8 servings
Exchange, 1 serving (without pastry shell): 1 fruit, 1 fat
Calories, 1 serving (without pastry shell): 120
Carbohydrates, 1 serving (without pastry shell): 15 g

Fresh Peach Cream Pie

	pastry shell, baked	
2 pkgs.	vanilla-flavored sugar-free	2 pkgs.
(4-serving)	to-cook pudding mix	(4-serving)
1 qt.	skim milk	1 L
1 t.	peach flavoring	5 mL
1 t.	grated lemon peel	5 mL
4	fresh peaches	4

Combine vanilla pudding mix, milk, peach flavoring, and lemon peel in a saucepan. Stir to dissolve pudding mix. Cook and stir over medium heat until mixture comes to a full boil. Set aside and allow to cool for 5 to 10 minutes. Pour into prepared pastry shell. Refrigerate until set. Meanwhile, remove pits from peaches and peel them. Slice each peach into 12 slices. Soak in lemon-juice water until ready to use. When filling is thoroughly set, remove peaches from lemon water, pat dry with paper towels, and arrange peach slices on top of pie. Refrigerate until ready to serve.

Yield: 8 servings
Exchange, 1 serving (without pastry shell): ½ skim milk, 1 fruit
Calories, 1 serving (without pastry shell): 95
Carbohydrates, 1 serving (without pastry shell): 17 g

Lime Fluff Pie

	pastry shell, baked	
1 pkg.	sugar-free lime gelatin	1 pkg.
(4-serving)		(4-serving)
1 pkg.	vanilla-flavored sugar-free	1 pkg.
(4-serving)	to-cook pudding mix	(4-serving)
2 c.	skim milk	500 mL

Prepare lime gelatin as directed on package. Pour into a medium-sized narrow bowl to chill. Refrigerate until completely set. Meanwhile, combine vanilla pudding mix and milk in a saucepan. Cook and stir over medium heat until mixture comes to a full boil. Cover and allow to cool. With an electric mixer, beat the set gelatin until frothy. Then beat the cooled pudding into the gelatin. Transfer mixture to prepared pie shell. Refrigerate until thoroughly set.

Yield: 8 servings
Exchange, 1 serving (without pastry shell): ⅓ bread
Calories, 1 serving (without pastry shell): 38
Carbohydrates, 1 serving (without pastry shell): 6 g

Sweet Cherry Coconut Pie

	baked pastry shell	
2 bags	Flavorland frozen dark sweet cherries	2 bags
(16-oz.)		(453-g)
¾ c.	water	190 mL
3 T.	cornstarch	45 mL
2 T.	granulated fructose	30 mL
1 t.	lemon juice	5 mL
3-oz. pkg.	cream cheese, room temperature	86-g pkg.
⅓ c.	unsweetened grated or shredded coconut, toasted	90 mL

Partially thaw cherries. Combine water, cornstarch, fructose, and lemon juice in a saucepan. Cook and stir over medium heat until mixture is a very thick paste. Remove from heat and fold in cherries until all cherries are coated and mixture is clear. Set aside to cool. Spread softened cream cheese on the bottom of the baked pastry shell. Sprinkle with the toasted coconut. Press the coconut slightly into the cheese. Transfer sweet cherry mixture to the shell and arrange evenly. If desired, decorate with pastry cutouts. Chill thoroughly.

Yield: 8 servings
Exchange, 1 serving (without pastry shell): 1½ fruit, ¾ fat
Calories, 1 serving (without pastry shell): 133
Carbohydrates, 1 serving (without pastry shell): 22 g

Chocolate Cherry Pie

	pastry shell, baked*	
16-oz. bag	Flavorland frozen dark sweet cherries, thawed	453-g bag
1 T.	cornstarch	15 mL
2 c.	skim milk	500 mL
3 T.	granulated fructose	45 mL
3 T.	unsweetened cocoa powder	45 mL
3 T.	all-purpose flour	45 mL
1 T.	vegetable oil	15 mL
1 t.	vanilla flavoring	5 mL
dash	salt	dash

*This pie is good with a chocolate crumb crust.

Combine cherries and cornstarch in a large microwave bowl or saucepan. Microwave on HIGH for 3 to 4 minutes or cook over medium heat until liquid is clear and thickened. Cover and allow to cool. Combine remaining ingredients in a large microwave measuring cup or bowl or in a saucepan. Stir to completely blend.

Microwave: Cook on HIGH for 5 minutes; then stir and continue cooking on MEDIUM 5 to 8 more minutes, stirring after every 3 minutes, until mixture is thick. Cover and cool to room temperature.

On top of stove: Stirring, cook over medium heat until mixture comes to a full boil. Reduce heat and cook until mixture is thick. Cover and cool to room temperature.

Transfer half of the cooled cherry mixture to the bottom of the pastry shell. Pour chocolate pudding in shell and spread evenly. Carefully spoon remaining cherry mixture over chocolate pudding. Chill until thoroughly set.

Yield: 8 servings
Exchange, 1 serving (without pastry shell): 1 fruit, ¼ bread
Calories, 1 serving (without pastry shell): 78
Carbohydrates, 1 serving (without pastry shell): 15 g

Red Raspberry Pie

	baked pastry shell	
1 qt.	frozen unsweetened red raspberries	1 L
1 c.	water	250 mL
3 T.	cornstarch	45 mL
⅓ c.	granulated fructose	90 mL
2 t.	lemon juice	10 mL
3-oz. pkg.	cream cheese, room temperature	86-g pkg.
1 T.	skim milk	15 mL

Partially thaw red raspberries. Combine water, cornstarch, fructose, and lemon juice in a saucepan. Cook and stir over medium heat until mixture is very thick. Fold partially frozen raspberries into mixture until all berries are coated and mixture is evenly distributed throughout the berries. Set aside to cool. Combine cream cheese and milk, and beat to blend. Spread cream cheese mixture over bottom of baked pastry shell. Spread cooled berry mixture over cream cheese mixture. Chill until firm. If desired, serve with a dot of nondairy whipped topping on each piece of pie.

Yield: 8 servings
Exchange, 1 serving (without pastry shell): ¾ fruit, ¾ fat
Calories, 1 serving (without pastry shell): 96
Carbohydrates, 1 serving (without pastry shell): 11 g

Chocolate Raspberry Pie

	pastry shell, baked*	
2 pkgs.	chocolate-flavored sugar-free	2 pkgs.
(4-serving)	to-cook pudding mix	(4-serving)
1 qt.	skim milk	1 L
2 c.	fresh raspberries	500 mL

*This pie is good with a cracker crumb crust.

Combine chocolate pudding mix and milk in a saucepan. Cook and stir over medium heat until mixture comes to a full boil. Allow to cool for 5 to 10 minutes or until pan can comfortably be held. Fold in raspberries. Transfer to pastry shell. Chill until thoroughly set and ready to serve.

Yield: 8 servings
Exchange, 1 serving (without pastry shell): ¾ skim milk, ¼ fruit
Calories, 1 serving (without pastry shell): 93
Carbohydrates, 1 serving (without pastry shell): 16 g

Peach Blueberry Pie

	pastry shell, baked*	
1 pkg.	vanilla-flavored sugar-free	1 pkg.
(4-serving)	to-cook pudding mix	(4-serving)
1 t.	almond flavoring	5 mL
2 c.	sliced fresh peaches	500 mL
	juice of 1 lemon	
2 c.	cleaned fresh blueberries	500 mL

*This pie is good with a graham cracker or meringue crust.

Prepare vanilla pudding mix as directed on package for pie, adding the almond flavoring. Allow to cool for 5 to 10 minutes. Pour filling into prepared pastry shell. Chill until set. Just before serving, sprinkle peaches with lemon juice. Arrange peaches and blueberries on pie. Chill until serving time.

Yield: 8 servings
Exchange, 1 serving (without pastry shell): 1 fruit
Calories, 1 serving (without pastry shell): 54
Carbohydrates, 1 serving (without pastry shell): 13 g

Chocolate Brandy Pecan Pie

	pastry shell, baked*	
2 pkgs.	chocolate-flavored sugar-free	2 pkgs.
(4-serving)	to-cook pudding mix	(4-serving)
1 qt.	skim milk	1 L
2 T.	brandy	30 mL
½ t.	vanilla flavoring	2 mL
½ c.	pecan halves	125 mL

*This pie is good with a chocolate crumb crust.

Combine chocolate pudding mix and milk in a saucepan. Cook and stir over medium heat until mixture comes to a full boil. Remove from heat; then stir in brandy and vanilla flavoring. Allow to cool for 5 to 10 minutes. Transfer to pastry shell. Decorate with pecan halves. Chill until thoroughly set.

Yield: 8 servings
Exchange, 1 serving (without pastry shell): 1 bread, 1 fat
Calories, 1 serving (without pastry shell): 126
Carbohydrates, 1 serving (without pastry shell): 13 g

Butterscotch Pie

	pastry shell, baked*	
1 pkg.	chocolate-flavored sugar-free	1 pkg.
(4-serving)	to-cook pudding mix	(4-serving)
1 qt.	skim milk	1 L
1 pkg.	butterscotch-flavored sugar-free	1 pkg.
(4-serving)	instant pudding mix	(4-serving)

*This pie is good with a graham cracker crust.

Combine chocolate pudding mix and 2 c. (500 mL) of milk in a saucepan. Cook and stir over medium heat until mixture comes to a full boil. Set aside and allow to cool for 5 to 10 minutes. Combine butterscotch pudding and the remaining 2 c. (500 mL) of milk in a second saucepan. Cook and stir over medium heat until mixture comes to a full boil. Set aside and cool for 5 to 10 minutes. Pour half of the butterscotch mixture into the bottom of the prepared pastry shell. Refrigerate until set. Pour all of the chocolate pudding on top of the butterscotch pudding in the pie shell. Cover with remaining butterscotch pudding. Chill until completely set.

Yield: 8 servings
Exchange, 1 serving (without pastry shell): 1 skim milk
Calories, 1 serving (without pastry shell): 75
Carbohydrates, 1 serving (without pastry shell): 12 g

Apple and Raisin Pie

	pastry shell, unbaked	
20-oz. can	unsweetened sliced apples	567-g can
½ c.	raisins	125 mL
3 T.	Cary's Sugar-Free Maple-Flavored Syrup	45 mL
1½ t.	all-purpose flour	7 mL
½ t.	ground cinnamon	2 mL

Combine sliced apples, raisins, syrup, flour, and cinnamon in a bowl. Fold to blend ingredients. Transfer to the pastry shell. Bake at 450 °F (230 °C) for 10 minutes; then reduce heat to 350 °F (175 °C) and continue baking for 30 more minutes or until set.

Yield: 8 servings
Exchange, 1 serving (without pastry shell): 1 fruit
Calories, 1 serving (without pastry shell): 58
Carbohydrates, 1 serving (without pastry shell): 16 g

Chocolate Chip Mint Cream Pie

	pastry shell, baked	
2 pkgs.	vanilla-flavored sugar-free	2 pkgs.
(4-serving)	to-cook pudding mix	(4-serving)
1 qt.	skim milk	1 L
1½ t.	peppermint flavoring	7 mL
4 drops	green food coloring	4 drops
¼ c.	mini–chocolate chips	60 mL
1 c.	prepared nondairy whipped topping	250 mL

Combine vanilla pudding mix, milk, flavoring, and food coloring in a saucepan. Stir to dissolve pudding mix. Cook and stir over medium heat until mixture comes to a full boil. Set aside and allow to cool. Fold in chocolate chips. Transfer to prepared pastry shell. Refrigerate until set. Decorate with nondairy whipped topping. Refrigerate until ready to serve.

Yield: 8 servings
Exchange, 1 serving (without pastry shell): 1 skim milk, ¾ fat
Calories, 1 serving (without pastry shell): 124
Carbohydrates, 1 serving (without pastry shell): 17 g

Plain Custard Pie

	unbaked pastry shell	
4	eggs, slightly beaten	4
¼ t.	salt	1 mL
¼ c.	granulated fructose	60 mL
3 c.	skim milk	750 mL
1 t.	vanilla flavoring or extract	5 mL
	ground nutmeg	

Combine eggs, salt, and fructose in a mixing bowl. Beat with a wire whisk or fork until thoroughly blended. Beat in skim milk and vanilla flavoring. Pour into unbaked pastry shell. Sprinkle with nutmeg. Bake at 425 °F (220 °C) for 10 minutes. Reduce heat to 300 °F (150 °C) and continue baking for 30 to 40 more minutes or until knife inserted in middle comes out clean.

Yield: 8 servings
Exchange, 1 serving (without pastry shell): ⅔ skim milk, 1 fat
Calories, 1 serving (without pastry shell): 86
Carbohydrates, 1 serving (without pastry shell): 8 g

Cool Strawberry Pie

	pastry shell, baked	
1 pkg.	sugar-free strawberry gelatin	1 pkg.
(4-serving)		(4-serving)
1 qt.	fresh strawberries, rinsed and hulled	1 L

Prepare gelatin as directed on package. Cool until gelatin resembles a thick syrup. Arrange strawberries in the pastry shell. Spoon thickened gelatin over the top. Refrigerate until thoroughly set.

Yield: 8 servings
Exchange, 1 serving (without pastry shell): ⅓ fruit
Calories, 1 serving (without pastry shell): 22
Carbohydrates, 1 serving (without pastry shell): 5 g

Apple Pie

	pastry shell, unbaked	
20-oz. can	unsweetened sliced apples	567-g can
1½ t.	apple-pie spice	7 mL
2 T.	cornstarch	30 mL
1 T.	granulated sugar replacement	15 mL
1 t.	apple flavoring	5 mL
½ t.	vanilla flavoring	2 mL
1 t.	powdered butter flavoring	5 mL
½ c.	corn flakes, finely crushed	125 mL

Drain liquid from sliced apples into a measuring cup. Transfer drained apple slices to the pastry shell. Sprinkle with apple-pie spice. Add enough water to the sliced-apples liquid to make ¼ c. (60 mL) of liquid. Stir in cornstarch until it is dissolved. Add sugar replacement, apple flavoring, and vanilla flavoring. Pour over apple slices in pastry shell. Sprinkle with powdered butter flavoring and crushed corn flakes. Bake at 425 °F (220 °C) for 30 minutes.

Yield: 8 servings
Exchange, 1 serving (without pastry shell): ⅔ fruit
Calories, 1 serving (without pastry shell): 37
Carbohydrates, 1 serving (without pastry shell): 9 g

Milk-Chocolate Chiffon Pie

	baked pastry shell	
¼ c.	cold water	60 mL
1 c.	skim milk	250 mL
1 env.	unflavored gelatin	1 env.
⅓ c.	carob powder	90 mL
dash	salt	dash
3	eggs	3
2 T.	granulated sugar replacement	30 mL
2 T.	granulated fructose	30 mL
1 t.	vanilla flavoring or extract	5 mL
1 t.	chocolate flavoring	5 mL
2 T.	granulated sugar replacement	30 mL
1 c.	prepared nondairy whipped topping	250 mL

Combine cold water and milk in a saucepan or large microwave bowl. Stir in gelatin, carob powder, and salt. On top of stove, cook and stir over medium heat until gelatin and carob powder are dissolved. Remove from heat. Or, in microwave, cook on MEDIUM-HIGH for 1 minute; then stir to dissolve gelatin and carob powder. Separate eggs. Place egg yolks in a measuring cup, egg whites in a mixing bowl. Beat egg yolks slightly with a fork; then add the 2 T. (30 mL) of sugar replacement and the fructose and flavorings to beaten egg yolks. Stir to completely mix. Stir into carob mixture. Cook on MEDIUM either on top of stove or in microwave until mixture starts to thicken. Stir and allow to cool. Meanwhile, beat egg whites into light peaks, and gradually add the 2 T. (30 mL) of sugar replacement. Beat into stiff peaks. Fold into chilled chocolate mixture. Fold nondairy whipped topping into chocolate mixture. Transfer to baked pastry shell. Chill until set, about 3 hours.

Yield: 8 servings
Exchange, 1 serving (without pastry shell): ½ bread, 1 fat
Calories, 1 serving (without pastry shell): 88
Carbohydrates, 1 serving (without pastry shell): 9 g

Tarts & Tortes

Tarts are special little pies, while tortes are considered elaborate cakes. With the introduction of ready-to-use pastry sheets, sticks, and boxed crumbs, tarts are easy to make. Tarts and tortes might be called the more creative side of pastry making. With tarts, you can create beautiful designs with the fruits and nuts. These open-faced "pies" are made in flat pans that lend themselves to making all kinds of wonderfully imaginative desserts. After you get started, you might want to check at your local kitchen specialty shop for different styles of tart and torte pans. I have used the very basic round pan for most of these recipes, but the same amount of dough can fit into many different pan shapes.

Tortes are the fun extension of cakes. Many of the tortes are simply cakes cut into many layers, then filled and the layers replaced. Here again, your choice of color and texture will make a dramatic difference in both the appearance and flavor of the torte.

Applesauce Tart

8 or 9 in.	flat pastry sheet	20 or 23 cm
3 T.	granulated fructose	45 mL
3 T.	margarine	45 mL
2 t.	rum flavoring	10 mL
2 c.	unsweetened applesauce	500 mL
2	firm MacIntosh apples	2

Place pastry sheet in a removable-bottom 8- or 9-in. (20- or 23-cm) tart pan. Prick sides and bottom many times with a fork. Bake at 375 °F (190 °C) for 15 to 18 minutes or until golden brown. Cool completely before filling. Combine fructose, rum flavoring, and margarine in a heavy or nonstick saucepan. Cook over low heat until fructose is dissolved. Stir in applesauce and

88

heat thoroughly. Meanwhile, core the apples and cut into as many very thin slices as possible. Put the applesauce-sauce filling into the baked tart shell. Arrange the apple slices around edge of tart. Bake at 400 °F (200 °C) for about 10 minutes or until apples are soft and edges begin to curl. If desired, sprinkle apple slices with a small amount of ground cinnamon before baking.

Yield: 8 servings
Exchange, 1 serving: 1 bread, 1 fruit, 2 fat
Calories, 1 serving: 227
Carbohydrates, 1 serving: 30 g

Pineapple Cream Tart

9 in.	baked tart shell, cooled	23 cm
1 c.	skim milk	250 mL
2 T.	granulated fructose	30 mL
1 T.	cornstarch	15 mL
3-oz. pkg.	cream cheese	86-g pkg.
20-oz. can	pineapple rings in juice	567-g can
1 env.	unflavored gelatin	1 env.

Combine milk, fructose, and cornstarch in a small saucepan. Cook and stir over medium heat until thick. Cut cream cheese into smaller pieces. Stir into hot mixture. Cool completely. Meanwhile, drain as much liquid from the pineapple rings as possible. If needed, add enough water to make 1½ c. (375 mL) of liquid. Sprinkle gelatin on top of liquid. Allow to soften; then heat to boiling and stir to dissolve gelatin. Cool until almost set but still in semiliquid state. While cream cheese mixture and pineapple-liquid mixture are cooling, place pineapple rings on paper towels to drain. Spread cream cheese mixture, when cool, into bottom of prepared tart shell. Chill until almost set. Arrange drained pineapple rings around edge of tart, overlapping where necessary. Cut any remaining pineapple rings into pieces that will fit in middle or other places in the design. Refrigerate tart until gelatin is partially set. Then spread partially set gelatin over entire surface of tart. Chill completely.

Yield: 8 servings
Exchange, 1 serving: 1 bread, 1 fruit, 1 fat
Calories, 1 serving: 205
Carbohydrates, 1 serving: 30 g

Mandarin Orange Parfait Tart

9 in.	baked tart shell	23 cm
2 cans	mandarin orange sections in water	2 cans
(15-oz.)		(425-g)
1 pkg.	sugar-free orange gelatin	1 pkg.
(4-serving)		(4-serving)
½ c.	cold water	125 mL
2 c.	calorie-reduced vanilla ice cream	500 mL

Drain liquid from both cans of mandarin oranges into a measuring cup (if needed, add water) to make 1 c. (250 mL) of liquid. Place orange sections in a strainer and allow to continue draining. Heat orange liquid to boiling; then stir in gelatin until dissolved. Remove from heat. Stir in the ½ c. (125 mL) of cold water. Add ice cream by spoonfuls to hot orange liquid. Stir until ice cream is completely melted. Chill until mixture is partially set or mixture mounds slightly when dropped from a spoon. Remove 10 to 15 mandarin orange sections from drained oranges. Set aside. Fold remaining orange sections into gelatin–ice cream mixture. Transfer to baked tart shell. Chill until set. Decorate top with reserved mandarin orange sections.

Yield: 8 servings
Exchange, 1 serving: 1 bread, ½ low-fat milk, 1 fat
Calories, 1 serving: 196
Carbohydrates, 1 serving: 25 g

Lemon Walnut Tart

9 in.	unbaked tart shell	23 cm
½ c.	finely chopped English walnuts	125 mL
3	eggs	3
⅓ c.	granulated fructose	90 mL
2 T.	granulated sugar replacement	30 mL
¼ c.	lemon juice	60 mL
1½ T.	grated lemon peel	21 mL
¾ t.	baking powder	7 mL
¼ t.	ground cloves	1 mL
dash	salt	dash
8 large	fresh strawberries, cleaned	8 large

Sprinkle chopped walnuts on the bottom of the unbaked tart shell. Combine eggs, fructose, sugar replacement, lemon juice, lemon peel, baking powder, cloves, and salt in a mixing bowl. Beat to blend thoroughly. Pour mixture over the nut base. Bake at 350 °F (175 °C) for 30 to 35 minutes or until middle is set. Cool completely. Just before serving, cut four or five slices down from tip of each strawberry nearly to the base. Fan out each strawberry and lay decoratively around the edge of the tart.

Yield: 8 servings
Exchange, 1 serving: 1 bread, ⅓ fruit, 2 fat
Calories, 1 serving: 158
Carbohydrates, 1 serving: 21 g

Canned Pear Tart

8 or 9 in.	flat pastry sheet	20 or 23 cm
⅓ c.	margarine, softened	90 mL
¼ c.	granulated fructose	60 mL
1	egg	1
⅓ c.	finely ground almonds	90 mL
1 T.	rum flavoring	15 mL
1 t.	almond flavoring	5 mL
1 T.	all-purpose flour	15 mL
2 cans	pear halves in juice	2 cans
(1-lb.)		(454-g)

Place pastry sheet in a removable-bottom 8- or 9-in. (20- or 23-cm) tart pan. Chill. Whip margarine and fructose until fluffy. Add egg, ground almonds, rum, and almond flavoring. Beat thoroughly. Beat in flour. Spread the mixture on the bottom of the chilled tart shell. Place back in refrigerator. Open and drain pears, reserving liquid in a small saucepan. Place each half, cut side down, on a cutting board. Slice each half crosswise into thin slices. Arrange the sliced pear halves around the edge of the tart, on top of filling. Place extra sliced pear halves decoratively in middle of tart. Bake at 400 °F (200 °C) for 30 to 40 minutes or until tart shell is golden. Meanwhile, bring the reserved pear liquid to a boil, reduce heat, and continue cooking until liquid is about ¼ c. (60 mL). Brush this liquid over the hot pears in the tart.

Yield: 8 servings
Exchange, 1 serving: 1 bread, 1 fruit, 2 fat
Calories, 1 serving: 300
Carbohydrates, 1 serving: 34 g

Coffee Cinnamon Tart

9 in.	unbaked tart shell, chilled	23 cm
2 T.	instant coffee powder	30 mL
2 T.	water	30 mL
3	eggs	3
¼ c.	granulated fructose	60 mL
2 T.	granulated sugar replacement	30 mL
¼ t.	ground cinnamon	1 mL
dash	salt	dash
8 T.	prepared nondairy whipped topping	120 mL

Dissolve coffee powder in the water. Combine eggs, fructose, sugar replacement, cinnamon, and salt in a mixing bowl. Beat to blend thoroughly. Beat in coffee water. Pour mixture into prepared tart shell. Bake at 350 °F (175 °C) for 25 to 30 minutes or until middle is set. Cool completely. Just before serving, place 1 T. (15 mL) of nondairy whipped topping on each piece.

Yield: 8 servings
Exchange, 1 serving: 1 bread, 1½ fat
Calories, 1 serving: 166
Carbohydrates, 1 serving: 18 g

Peach Parfait Tart

9 in.	baked tart shell	23 cm
29-oz. can	sliced peaches in juice	822-g can
1 pkg. (4-serving)	sugar-free lemon gelatin	1 pkg. (4-serving)
½ c.	cold water	125 mL
2 c.	calorie-reduced vanilla ice cream	500 mL

Drain peaches, reserving liquid. Add enough water to the peach liquid to make 1 c. (250 mL). Heat to boiling; then stir in gelatin until dissolved. Add the cold water. Remove from heat. Add ice cream by spoonfuls to hot liquid. Stir until ice cream is completely melted. Chill until mixture is partially set or mixture mounds slightly when dropped from a spoon. Turn into baked tart shell. Chill until set. Decorate with peach slices.

Yield: 8 servings
Exchange, 1 serving: 1 bread, ½ low-fat milk, ½ fruit, 1 fat
Calories, 1 serving: 234
Carbohydrates, 1 serving: 35 g

Fresh Apple Tart

9 in.	unbaked tart shell	23 cm
8	Cortland or Rome apples	8
1 t.	cornstarch	5 mL
1 t.	water	5 mL
1	egg	1
¼ c.	Cary's Sugar-Free Maple-Flavored Syrup	60 mL

Core the apples and cut in half; don't peel. Place one apple half in middle of unbaked tart shell. Place remaining halves around edge of shell. If you have any extra apple halves, slice and place decoratively in the design. Dissolve the cornstarch in the water in a small cup. Add egg and beat with a fork until completely blended. Stir in maple syrup. Pour over apples. Bake at 425 °F (220 °C) for 30 minutes; reduce heat to 350 °F (175 °C) and continue baking another 15 minutes. Serve hot or cold.

Yield: 8 servings
Exchange, 1 serving: 1 bread, 1 fruit, 1 fat
Calories, 1 serving: 232
Carbohydrates, 1 serving: 31 g

Single Strawberry Tart

1	baked individual tart shell	1
½ c.	sugar-free frozen strawberries	125 mL
1 t.	granulated fructose	5 mL
1 t.	cornstarch	5 mL
2 t.	water	10 mL

Place strawberries in a microwave bowl or cup. Cook on HIGH in the microwave for 30 seconds. Dissolve fructose and cornstarch in the water in a small cup. Pour into warmed strawberries. Microwave on HIGH for 1 minute more, stirring after 30 seconds. Stir and allow to cool. If liquid is not clear, return to microwave and cook 15 seconds more or until mixture is clear. Allow to cool. Transfer to baked individual tart shell. If desired, top with 1 T. of prepared nondairy whipped topping. (This tart is perfect for a Valentine's Day gift.)

Yield: 1 serving
Exchange, 1 serving: 1 bread, ⅓ fruit, 1 fat
Calories, 1 serving: 145
Carbohydrates, 1 serving: 20 g

Fresh Strawberry Tart

9 in.	baked tart shell	23 cm
1 c.	prepared nondairy whipped topping	250 mL
3 c.	fresh strawberries, cleaned	750 mL

Spoon nondairy whipped topping into tart shell and arrange strawberries on top, stem side down. Chill thoroughly. If desired, decorate with a few of the strawberry greens to add contrast of color. Remove greens when serving.

Yield: 8 servings
Exchange, 1 serving: 1 bread, ½ fruit, 1 fat
Calories, 1 serving: 158
Carbohydrates, 1 serving: 21 g

Kiwi Cream Tart

9 in.	baked tart shell	23 cm
1 box	vanilla-flavored sugar-free	1 box
(4-serving)	to-cook pudding mix	(4-serving)
9	kiwis	9

Prepare vanilla pudding mix as directed on package for pie. Spoon into baked tart shell. Refrigerate until set. Peel kiwis and slice eight of the kiwis lengthwise almost to the bottom. Fan each kiwi from the bottom and lay around edge of tart. Slice the remaining kiwi lengthwise into thin slices. Lay these slices around the middle of the tart, overlapping if needed.

Yield: 8 servings
Exchange, 1 serving: 1½ bread, 1 fruit, 1 fat
Calories, 1 serving: 225
Carbohydrates, 1 serving: 37 g

Easy Chocolate Tart

9 in.	baked tart shell	23 cm
1 box	chocolate-flavored sugar-free	1 box
(4-serving)	to-cook pudding mix	(4-serving)
1½ c.	prepared nondairy whipped topping	375 mL
	mint leaves (optional)	

Prepare chocolate pudding mix as directed on package for pie. Allow to thicken; then fold in 1 c. (250 mL) of the nondairy whipped topping. Pile into baked tart shell. Drop four or five mounds of the remaining topping on top of tart. With a fork, swirl into the tart for a design. Chill thoroughly before serving. Garnish with mint leaves.

Yield: 8 servings
Exchange, 1 serving: 1½ bread, 1½ fat
Calories, 1 serving: 194
Carbohydrates, 1 serving: 23 g

Easy Raspberry Tart for a Crowd

Crust

½ c.	margarine	125 mL
¼ c.	granulated sugar replacement	60 mL
1	egg	1
1 T.	grated lemon peel	15 mL
1 c.	all-purpose flour	250 mL
½ t.	baking powder	2 mL

Filling

1 pkg. (4-serving)	sugar-free raspberry gelatin	1 pkg. (4-serving)
1½ c.	boiling water	375 mL
1 qt.	fresh whole raspberries, cleaned	1 mL

For crust: Beat margarine and sugar replacement until light. Beat in the egg and lemon peel. Combine flour and baking powder in a bowl. Gradually beat into creamed mixture; then beat until smooth. Line a 9 × 12 in. (23 × 30 cm) pan with wax paper. Spray paper with a vegetable spray. Spread dough evenly onto it. Bake at 375 °F (190 °C) for 15 to 20 minutes or until lightly browned. Chill thoroughly.

For filling: Dissolve the raspberry gelatin in the boiling water. Chill until syrupy. Spread about a third of the cooled gelatin on top of the chilled crust. Arrange raspberries on top of the gelatin. Spoon remaining gelatin evenly over the fruit. Chill until set.

Yield: 24 servings
Exchange, 1 serving: ⅓ fruit, 1 fat
Calories, 1 serving: 67
Carbohydrates, 1 serving: 4 g

Fresh Blueberry Glazed Tart

9 in.	baked tart shell	23 cm
3-oz. pkg.	cream cheese, softened	86-g pkg.
2 c.	fresh blueberries, cleaned	500 mL
¼ c.	all-natural blueberry preserves	60 mL

Whip cream cheese until very creamy. Spread on the bottom of the baked tart shell. Arrange blueberries in a single layer on top of cheese. Melt preserves and pour over blueberries. Refrigerate.

Yield: 8 servings
Exchange, 1 serving: 1 bread, 1 fruit, 1 fat
Calories, 1 serving: 174
Carbohydrates, 1 serving: 25 g

Pretty Pear Tart

9 in.	baked tart shell	23 cm
2 cans	pear halves in juice	2 cans
(1-lb.)		(456-g)
2 t.	cornstarch	10 mL

Completely drain pear halves, reserving ¾ c. (190 mL) of liquid. Decoratively lay pear halves in the baked tart shell. Combine reserved pear liquid and cornstarch in a bowl or saucepan. Cook on HIGH in microwave for 30 to 40 seconds or on top of stove, until liquid is clear and thickened. Pour over pears. Bake at 400 °F (200 °C) for 15 to 20 minutes or until pears look slightly glazed and baked. Serve hot or cold.

Yield: 8 servings
Exchange, 1 serving: 1 bread, 1 fruit, 1 fat
Calories, 1 serving: 202
Carbohydrates, 1 serving: 29 g

Almond Cream Torte

1 c.	vanilla wafer crumbs	250 mL
3 T.	melted margarine	45 mL
2 T.	cold water	30 mL
1 env.	unflavored gelatin	1 env.
1 pkg.	vanilla-flavored sugar-free	1 pkg.
(4-serving)	to-cook pudding mix	(4-serving)

1 t.	vanilla flavoring or extract	5 mL
½ t.	almond extract	2 mL
¼ c.	ground almonds	60 mL

Combine wafer crumbs and melted margarine in a bowl. Using a fork, stir to blend. Press mixture into the bottom and sides of a 9-in. (23-cm) lightly greased round pan to form a crust. Place in freezer to chill. Combine cold water and gelatin in a small cup. Allow to soften. Meanwhile, prepare vanilla pudding mix as directed on package for pie. Remove from heat; then add softened gelatin, vanilla, and almond extract. Stir until gelatin is dissolved. Chill thoroughly but not until fully set. Stir in ground almonds. Pour into chilled crust. Refrigerate.

Yield: 10 servings
Exchange, 1 serving: 1 bread, 1½ fat
Calories, 1 serving: 110
Carbohydrates, 1 serving: 10 g

One-Layer Blitz Torte

8-oz. pkg.	sugar-free yellow cake mix	226-g pkg.
2	egg whites	2
2 T.	granulated sugar replacement	30 mL
¼ t.	vanilla flavoring or extract	1 mL
⅛ t.	cream of tartar	½ mL
¼ c.	sliced almonds	60 mL
1 pkg. (4-serving)	vanilla-flavored sugar-free instant pudding mix, prepared	1 pkg. (4-serving)

Prepare cake mix as directed on package. Place a piece of wax paper on the bottom of an 8-in. (20-cm) round cake pan. Transfer cake batter to pan. Combine egg whites, sugar replacement, vanilla, and cream of tartar in a narrow mixing bowl. Beat until very stiff peaks form, for about 5 minutes. Spread over cake mix in pan. Sprinkle surface with almonds. Preheat oven to 425 °F (220 °C). Place cake in oven and reduce heat to 350 °F (175 °C). Bake for 25 to 30 minutes. Cool completely. Frost top with prepared vanilla pudding. Serve.

Yield: 10 servings
Exchange, 1 serving: 1 bread, 1 fat
Calories, 1 serving: 112
Carbohydrates, 1 serving: 12 g

Strawberry Kiwi Torte

1 c.	vanilla wafer crumbs	250 mL
3 T.	melted margarine	45 mL
2 c.	prepared nondairy whipped topping	500 mL
1 qt.	fresh strawberries, cleaned and sliced*	1 L
4	kiwis, cleaned and sliced	4

*If desired, reserve a few of the strawberries whole for extra garnish around the plate.

Combine wafer crumbs and melted margarine in a bowl. Using a fork, stir to blend. Press mixture into the bottom and sides of an 8-in. (20-cm) lightly greased round pan to form a crust. Place in freezer to chill. Shortly before serving, spread a thin layer of nondairy whipped topping on the bottom of the crust. Place about half of the strawberry slices on top of the layer of whipped topping. Spread the remaining whipped topping over the strawberries. Decorate the top of the torte with the remaining strawberry and kiwi slices. Refrigerate.

Yield: 10 servings
Exchange, 1 serving: ½ bread, ½ fruit, 1 fat
Calories, 1 serving: 116
Carbohydrates, 1 serving: 13 g

Orange Refrigerator Torte

8-oz. pkg.	sugar-free yellow cake mix	226-g pkg.
¾ c.	orange juice, warmed slightly	190 mL
1 t.	grated lemon peel	5 mL
1 t.	grated orange peel	5 mL
½ t.	dry yeast	2 mL
15-oz. can	mandarin orange sections in water	425-g can
1 env.	unflavored gelatin	1 env.
2 c.	prepared nondairy whipped topping	500 mL

Combine yellow cake mix, orange juice, lemon and orange peel, and yeast in a mixing bowl. Beat well to blend. Transfer to 9-in.- (23-cm-) square greased-and-floured cake pan. Bake as directed on package. Meanwhile, drain mandarin orange liquid into a measuring cup; reserve orange sections. Add enough water to the orange liquid to make 1 c. (250 mL). Sprinkle gelatin over top of liquid and allow to soften for 1 to 2 minutes. Pour liquid into a saucepan and heat, stirring until gelatin is dissolved. Set aside to cool. When cake is baked, remove from pan and cool completely. Cut cake into three thin layers. Cut one layer in half. Place one-and-one-half layers on the bottom of a 9 × 12 in. (23 × 30 cm) pan. Fold cool gelatin mixture into nondairy whipped topping. Spread about a third of this mixture onto the layer of cake in pan. Place second layer and one-half onto the top of the whipped topping. Cover with remaining whipped topping mixture. Place cover or foil over cake and refrigerate until the next day. Just before serving, space orange sections attractively around top edge of cake.

Yield: 10 servings
Exchange, 1 serving: ½ bread, 1 fat
Calories, 1 serving: 109
Carbohydrates, 1 serving: 7 g

Quick Baked Apple Turnovers

1 sheet	unbaked puff pastry	1 sheet
1-lb. can	unsweetened sliced apples	456-g can
2 t.	granulated fructose	10 mL
1 t.	ground cinnamon	5 mL
1	egg yolk, slightly beaten	1
2 T.	sugar-free white frosting mix	30 mL

Remove one sheet of puff pastry from carton. Allow to soften for 20 minutes; then unfold onto a lightly floured surface. Lightly flour top surface and roll into a 12-in. (30-cm) square. Cut into nine 4-in. (10-cm) squares. Slightly drain apples. Pour into a bowl; then add fructose and cinnamon. Stir or flip to coat the apple slices. Place a spoonful of apple slices in the middle of each 4 × 4 in. (10 × 10 cm) square. Lightly brush the edges of two sides of each square with the egg yolk. Fold edges without egg yolk over to seal on egg yolk edges. Place on water-sprayed cookie sheet. Chill for at least 20 minutes. Bake at 400 °F (200 °C) for 15 to 20 minutes or until golden brown. Allow to cool. Combine frosting mix and very small amount of water in a bowl. Stir until smooth. Drizzle over top of turnovers.

Yield: 9 servings
Exchange, 1 serving: 1 bread, ⅔ fruit, 1 fat
Calories, 1 serving: 171
Carbohydrates, 1 serving: 26 g

Pistachio Nut Torte

8-oz pkg.	sugar-free white cake mix	226-g pkg.
1 t.	rum flavoring	5 mL
¼ t.	dry yeast	1 mL
1 pkg.	pistachio-flavored sugar-free	1 pkg.
(4-serving)	instant pudding mix	(4-serving)
¼ c.	pistachio nuts, ground fine	60 mL

Combine cake mix, rum flavoring, and dry yeast in a mixing bowl. Continue preparing cake mix as directed on package. Transfer to an 8-in. (20-cm) round greased-and-floured cake pan. Bake as directed on package. Cool completely. Prepare pistachio pudding mix with skim milk as directed on package. Allow to set completely. To assemble: Cut cake in half horizontally. Spread half of the pudding between the layers. Top with remaining cake layer, cover with remaining pudding, and sprinkle with pistachio nuts. Chill thoroughly before serving.

Yield: 10 servings
Exchange, 1 serving: 1 bread, 1 fat
Calories, 1 serving: 113
Carbohydrates, 1 serving: 12 g

Pear Puff

1 sheet	unbaked puff pastry	1 sheet
4	firm pears	4
1 pkg.	unsweetened cherry drink mix	1 pkg.
2 t.	granulated fructose	10 mL
1 c.	warm water	250 mL
1	egg yolk, beaten	1

Remove one sheet of puff pastry from carton. Allow to soften for 20 minutes; then unfold onto a lightly floured surface. Lightly flour top surface and roll into a 13-in. (33-cm) square. Use a 4-in. (10-cm) tart ring or dough cutter to cut out six rounds. Fold remaining dough together and roll large enough to cut out two more rounds. Place on a water-sprayed large cookie sheet. Turn the sides of each round up slightly to form an edge. Place in refrigerator until ready to use. Carefully peel pear, cut in half lengthwise, and remove core. Place pear halves in a bowl. Combine cherry drink mix and fructose in a bowl or measuring cup. Add the warm water, stirring to dissolve mix and fructose. Pour over pears. If needed, add additional water to completely cover pears. Cover and allow to tint for at least an hour. If you want a brighter red color, allow to tint overnight in the refrigerator. To assemble: Remove pears from water and drain well; pat dry. Using a sharp knife, cut each pear half in four thin slices lengthwise. Slightly fan the pear half from the tip and lay in the middle of each dough round. Brush the exposed dough edges with the beaten egg yolk. Bake at 400 °F (200 °C) for 15 to 20 minutes or until pastry is puffed and golden brown. Serve warm.

Yield: 8 servings
Exchange, 1 serving: 1 bread, ⅓ fruit, 1 fat
Calories, 1 serving: 144
Carbohydrates, 1 serving: 21 g

Sweet Cherry Puff

1 sheet	unbaked puff pastry	1 sheet
1-lb. bag	frozen unsweetened sweet cherries, thawed	453-g bag
1 T.	cornstarch	15 mL
2 t.	granulated fructose	10 mL
1 t.	grated lemon peel	5 mL

Remove one sheet of puff pastry from carton. Allow to soften for 20 minutes; then unfold onto a lightly floured surface. Lightly flour top surface and roll into an 11 × 14 in. (28 × 35 cm) rectangle. Place on a water-sprayed large cookie sheet. Turn the sides up slightly to form an edge. Chill in refrigerator at least 20 minutes. Combine thawed cherries, cornstarch, fructose, and lemon peel in a bowl. Stir or flip to blend. Pour into chilled pastry shell. Arrange fruit evenly. Bake at 400 °F (200 °C) for 20 to 25 minutes or until edges are golden brown and cherries and liquid appear partially set. Cool slightly before cutting.

Yield: 10 servings
Exchange, 1 serving: 1 bread, ⅔ fruit, 1 fat
Calories, 1 serving: 181
Carbohydrates, 1 serving: 26 g

Refrigerator & Frozen Desserts

There is nothing quite like swirling a cool refreshing light dessert in your mouth on a hot summer day. For those of us who love to make and eat desserts, the most rewarding part is the control we can have over the freshness of the ingredients, the flavor, and the calories in these desserts. The refrigerator and frozen desserts presented here are composed primarily of fruits, low-calorie pudding, egg whites, gelatin, and nondairy whipped topping.

Because of their low-fat content, many of these desserts freeze very hard. So, when preparing them for family or friends, allow time for the dessert to thaw out somewhat before serving time or package it in individual portions. If you decide to freeze in individual portions, garnish with the fresh ingredients just before serving.

Banana Pecan Frozen Dessert

1 pt.	nonfat sugar-free vanilla frozen dessert, vanilla ice cream, or frozen vanilla yogurt	500 mL
1	very ripe banana, mashed	1
¼ c.	chopped pecans	60 mL

Allow frozen dessert to thaw slightly. Beat in the mashed banana and chopped pecans. Pack in a freezer container or bowl. Cover and freeze until firm.

Yield: 6 servings

For frozen dessert:

Exchange, 1 serving: ¾ bread
Calories, 1 serving: 58
Carbohydrates, 1 serving: 11 g

For ice cream:

Exchange, 1 serving: 1½ bread, ⅓ fat
Calories, 1 serving: 92
Carbohydrates, 1 serving: 22 g

For frozen yogurt:

Exchange, 1 serving: 1 bread
Calories, 1 serving: 72
Carbohydrates, 1 serving: 13 g

Maple-Flavored Frozen Dessert

1 pt.	nonfat sugar-free vanilla frozen dessert, vanilla ice cream, or vanilla frozen yogurt	500 mL
¼ c.	Cary's Sugar-Free Maple-Flavored Syrup	60 mL
½ t.	maple flavoring	2 mL
¼ t.	vanilla extract	1 mL

Allow frozen dessert to thaw slightly. Beat in the maple syrup and flavoring. Stir in vanilla extract. Pack in a freezer container or bowl. Cover and freeze until firm.

Yield: 6 servings

For frozen dessert:

Exchange, 1 serving: 1 bread, ¼ fat
Calories, 1 serving: 95
Carbohydrates, 1 serving: 15 g

For ice cream:

Exchange, 1 serving: 1½ bread, 1 fat
Calories, 1 serving: 139
Carbohydrates, 1 serving: 25 g

For frozen yogurt:

Exchange, 1 serving: 1 bread, ½ fat
Calories, 1 serving: 117
Carbohydrates, 1 serving: 16 g

Crisp-Mixture Frozen Dessert

2 t.	margarine	10 mL
¼ c.	cereal flakes, slightly crushed	60 mL
2 T.	chopped walnuts	30 mL
1 pt.	nonfat sugar-free vanilla frozen dessert, vanilla ice cream, or vanilla frozen yogurt	500 mL

Melt margarine in a small nonstick frying pan on low heat. Stir in cereal flakes and walnuts. Stir or toss to completely coat. Stir and cook about a minute. Remove from heat and cool completely. Allow frozen dessert to thaw slightly. Stir the cereal-nut mixture into the frozen dessert. Pack in a freezer container or bowl. Cover and freeze until firm.

Yield: 6 servings

For frozen dessert:

Exchange, 1 serving: 1 bread
Calories, 1 serving: 77
Carbohydrates, 1 serving: 11 g

For ice cream:

Exchange, 1 serving: 1¼ bread, 1½ fat
Calories, 1 serving: 122
Carbohydrates, 1 serving: 21 g

For frozen yogurt:

Exchange, 1 serving: ¾ bread, 1 fat
Calories, 1 serving: 100
Carbohydrates, 1 serving: 12 g

Spicy Cinnamon Frozen Dessert

1 pt.	nonfat sugar-free vanilla frozen dessert, vanilla ice cream, or vanilla frozen yogurt	500 mL
1 T.	granulated fructose	15 mL
1 t.	ground cinnamon	5 mL
½ t.	ground nutmeg	2 mL
¼ t.	ground cloves	1 mL

Allow frozen dessert to thaw slightly. Beat in fructose, cinnamon, nutmeg, and cloves. If desired, ½ t. (2 mL) of apple flavoring can be added. Pack in a freezer container or bowl. Cover and freeze until firm.

Yield: 6 servings

For frozen dessert:

Exchange, 1 serving: 1 bread
Calories, 1 serving: 74
Carbohydrates, 1 serving: 17 g

For ice cream:

Exchange, 1 serving: 1½ bread, 1⅓ fat
Calories, 1 serving: 139
Carbohydrates, 1 serving: 28 g

For frozen yogurt:

Exchange, 1 serving: 1 bread, ¼ fat
Calories, 1 serving: 97
Carbohydrates, 1 serving: 18 g

Prune Frozen Dessert

| 1 pt. | nonfat sugar-free vanilla frozen dessert, vanilla ice cream, or vanilla frozen yogurt | 500 mL |
| 4-oz. jar | baby prunes | 113-g jar |

Allow frozen dessert to thaw slightly. Beat in prune puree. Pack in a freezer container or bowl. Cover and freeze until firm.

Yield: 6 servings

For frozen dessert:

Exchange, 1 serving: ½ bread, ⅓ fruit
Calories, 1 serving: 60
Carbohydrates, 1 serving: 14 g

For ice cream:

Exchange, 1 serving: 1 bread, ½ fruit, 1 fat
Calories, 1 serving: 135
Carbohydrates, 1 serving: 24 g

For frozen yogurt:

Exchange, 1 serving: ¾ bread, ⅓ fat
Calories, 1 serving: 83
Carbohydrates, 1 serving: 15 g

Toasted-Hazelnut Frozen Dessert

| ½ c. | hazelnuts | 125 mL |
| 1 pt. | nonfat sugar-free vanilla frozen dessert, vanilla ice cream, or vanilla frozen yogurt | 500 mL |

Place hazelnuts in a single layer on a baking sheet. Bake at 350 °F (175 °C) for 15 minutes or until lightly toasted. Cool slightly and rub off the very loose skins. (It's not necessary to rub all the skin off.) Chop hazelnuts. Cool. Allow frozen dessert to thaw slightly. Mix hazelnuts into the frozen dessert. Pack in a freezer container or bowl. Cover and freeze until firm.

Yield: 6 servings

For frozen dessert:

Exchange, 1 serving: 1 bread, ½ fat
Calories, 1 serving: 105
Carbohydrates, 1 serving: 11 g

For ice cream:

Exchange, 1 serving: 1¼ bread, 2 fat
Calories, 1 serving: 150
Carbohydrates, 1 serving: 22 g

For frozen yogurt:

Exchange, 1 serving: 1 bread, 1½ fat
Calories, 1 serving: 128
Carbohydrates, 1 serving: 12 g

Frozen Dessert with Raspberry Grand Marnier Sauce

10-oz. bag	frozen red raspberries	250-g bag
1½ T.	Grand Marnier	21 mL
6 T.	prepared nondairy whipped topping	90 mL
1 pt.	nonfat sugar-free vanilla frozen dessert, vanilla ice cream, or vanilla frozen yogurt	500 mL

Thaw and drain raspberries. Select six of the best raspberries for garnish and refrigerate. Place remaining raspberries in a bowl, and carefully fold in Grand Marnier. Cover and chill thoroughly. To serve: Divide frozen dessert of your choice evenly between six serving glasses. Spoon raspberries and liqueur over frozen dessert. Top with 1 T. (15 mL) of the nondairy whipped topping. Garnish with reserved raspberries.

Yield: 6 servings

For frozen dessert:

Exchange, 1 serving: ¾ bread, ½ fruit
Calories, 1 serving: 86
Carbohydrates, 1 serving: 16 g

For ice cream:

Exchange, 1 serving: 1 bread, ½ fruit, 1 fat
Calories, 1 serving: 131
Carbohydrates, 1 serving: 27 g

For frozen yogurt:

Exchange, 1 serving: 1 bread, ½ fat
Calories, 1 serving: 109
Carbohydrates, 1 serving: 17 g

Apricot Creme

1-lb. can	apricot halves in juice	454-g can
4-oz. jar	baby apricots	113-g jar
2 c.	prepared nondairy whipped topping	500 mL

Drain apricot halves and place in a food processor or blender. Process to a semipuree stage. Transfer to a bowl; stir in baby-food apricot puree and 1 cup (250 mL) of the nondairy whipped topping. Freeze for 3 to 4 hours or overnight. Cut frozen apricot mixture into pieces, and reprocess in a food processor to a frozen slush. Occasionally, stop machine to push mixture down. Return to freezer and chill again. About 2 or 3 hours before serving, check hardness of mixture; if necessary, return to processor and process until smooth. To serve: Divide the mixture evenly between eight serving glasses. Top with remaining whipped topping.

Yield: 8 servings
Exchange, 1 serving: ½ fruit, 1 fat
Calories, 1 serving: 79
Carbohydrates, 1 serving: 12 g

Strawberry Ice Cake

14	graham cracker squares	14
¼ c.	melted margarine	60 mL
1 env.	unflavored gelatin	1 env.
¼ c.	cold water	60 mL
1 pkg. (4-serving)	sugar-free strawberry gelatin	1 pkg. (4-serving)
1 c.	boiling water	250 mL
2 c.	fresh strawberries	500 mL
2 c.	prepared nondairy whipped topping	500 mL
1	egg white, beaten stiff	1

Crush graham crackers into fine crumbs; then add margarine and stir to mix. Line bottom and sides of a 9-in. (23-cm) pie pan or springform pan with the crumb mixture. Sprinkle the unflavored gelatin over the top of the cold water. Allow to soften for several minutes. Dissolve strawberry gelatin in the boiling water. Stir unflavored gelatin into strawberry gelatin and stir to dissolve gelatin. Cool completely. Cut strawberries in half. Select 16 of the prettiest halves for garnish, and reserve. Fold strawberries and nondairy whipped topping into the gelatin mixture thoroughly. Fold in egg white, leaving a few white streaks. Transfer to crumb-lined pan. Refrigerate until set or overnight. To serve, remove from springform pan. Transfer to serving plate and decorate with reserved strawberry halves.

Yield: 10 servings
Exchange, 1 serving: 1 bread, 1 fat
Calories, 1 serving: 128
Carbohydrates, 1 serving: 11 g

Raspberries with Peach Sauce

16-oz. pkg.	frozen peach slices	454-g pkg.
3 T.	granulated fructose	45 mL
⅓ c.	cold water	90 mL
2 t.	lemon juice	10 mL
1 t.	vanilla extract	5 mL
½ c.	low-fat plain yogurt	125 mL
2 c.	fresh raspberries	500 mL

Combine frozen peach slices, fructose, water, lemon juice, and vanilla extract in a food processor. Process until mixture is a slush. Add yogurt and process until smooth. Arrange about two-thirds to three-fourths of the raspberries in four stemmed glasses or cups. Spoon the peach slush over the top of the raspberries. Garnish with remaining fresh raspberries.

Yield: 4 servings
Exchange, 1 serving: 1 fruit
Calories, 1 serving: 58
Carbohydrates, 1 serving: 15 g

Frozen Cottage Cheese Torte

14	graham cracker squares	14
¼ c.	melted margarine	60 mL
2 env.	unflavored gelatin	2 env.
½ c.	cold water	125 mL
2	eggs, separated	2
½ c.	granulated fructose	125 mL
¼ c.	granulated sugar replacement	60 mL
dash	salt	dash
½ c.	skim milk	125 mL
16-oz. carton	low-fat cottage cheese	454-g carton
½ t.	vanilla extract	2 mL
2 c.	prepared nondairy whipped topping	500 mL

Crush graham crackers into fine crumbs; then add margarine and stir to mix. Line bottom and sides of a 9-in. (23-cm) springform pan with the crumb mixture. Chill. Sprinkle gelatin over cold water and allow to soften for several minutes. Beat egg yolks slightly; then pour into nonstick saucepan or top of double boiler.. Stir in fructose, sugar replacement, salt, and milk. Cook and stir over medium heat until mixture is thick and coats a spoon. Cool. Stir in cottage cheese and vanilla extract. Beat cottage cheese mixture until light and fluffy. Beat egg whites until stiff. Fold egg whites into cottage cheese mixture. Fold nondairy whipped topping into cottage cheese mixture. Transfer to a graham crust. Freeze for 8 to 10 hours or overnight.

Yield: 10 servings
Exchange, 1 serving: 1 bread, 1 fat
Calories, 1 serving: 163
Carbohydrates, 1 serving: 16 g

Three Fruit Parfait

1 c.	frozen strawberries, thawed	250 mL
1 pt.	nonfat sugar-free dairy dessert (any flavor)	500 mL
1 c.	frozen blueberries, thawed	250 mL
1	banana, sliced thin	1

Distribute about two-thirds to three-fourths of the thawed strawberries between six stemmed glasses or cups. Distribute half of the dairy dessert equally between the glasses. Top each with ⅙ c. of the blueberries. Spoon remaining dairy dessert evenly into the glasses. Distribute the sliced banana between the glasses. Top with the reserved strawberries.

Yield: 6 servings
Exchange, 1 serving: 1 fruit
Calories, 1 serving: 63
Carbohydrates, 1 serving: 15 g

Sweet Cherry O'Lee

1½ c.	cold water	375 mL
1 T.	cornstarch	15 mL
¼ t.	vanilla extract	1 mL
1 t.	unsweetened cherry drink mix	5 mL
2 c.	vanilla ice cream	500 mL
2 c.	frozen sweet cherries, thawed	500 L

Combine cold water and cornstarch in a saucepan. Stir to dissolve cornstarch. Cook and stir over medium heat until mixture comes to a boil. Continue boiling for 3 minutes, stirring occasionally. Remove from heat, and stir in vanilla extract. Cool to lukewarm; then stir in cherry drink mix. Place ⅓ c. (90 mL) of ice cream in each of the six glasses. (Wine glasses are very pretty to use.) Top each with ⅓ c. (90 mL) of the thawed sweet cherries. Distribute the warm cherry sauce evenly between the glasses.

Yield: 6 servings
Exchange, 1 serving: 1 bread, ½ fat
Calories, 1 serving: 109
Carbohydrates, 1 serving: 17 g

Chocolate Fluff

1 c.	cold water	250 mL
2 T.	granulated fructose	30 mL
1 T.	cornstarch	15 mL
4	egg whites	4
1 pkg.	chocolate-flavored sugar-free	1 pkg.
(4-serving)	instant pudding mix	(4-serving)
2½ c.	cold skim milk	625 mL

Combine cold water, fructose, and cornstarch in a small saucepan. Stir to dissolve cornstarch. Cook and stir over medium heat until clear and thickened. Remove from heat and cool to lukewarm. Beat egg whites until almost stiff. Gradually add cool cornstarch mixture, beating well after each addition. Mixture will become very white and thickened. Transfer to a 9-in.- (23-cm-) square pan or dish. Freeze. Just before serving, combine chocolate pudding mix and milk in a medium-sized bowl. Beat on low speed until mixture begins to thicken. Cut frozen fluff into nine equal squares. When serving, distribute the pudding evenly over the top of each square.

Yield: 9 servings
Exchange, 1 serving: ½ skim milk, ⅓ fruit
Calories, 1 serving: 53
Carbohydrates, 1 serving: 8 g

Frosty 'nilla

4 c.	skim milk	1000 mL
¼ c.	granulated fructose	60 mL
1 t.	vanilla extract	5 mL

Combine ingredients in a mixing bowl or measuring cup. Stir to dissolve fructose. Pour into an ice cream maker. (I use a Donvier, finding it faster and easier than others.) Freeze as directed by ice cream–maker manufacturer. You can pack "Frosty 'nilla" in a freezer container for later use. It freezes very hard in a normal freezer. I usually keep any extra in the refrigerator freezer.

Yield: 8 servings
Exchange, 1 serving: ½ skim milk, ⅓ fruit
Calories, 1 serving: 57
Carbohydrates, 1 serving: 9 g

Summer Strawberry Blaster

1 pkg. (4-serving)	sugar-free strawberry gelatin	1 pkg. (4-serving)
1 c.	boiling water	250 mL
1 c.	cold skim milk	250 mL

Dissolve the strawberry gelatin in the boiling water. Allow to cool to lukewarm. Stir in cold skim milk. (If water is hot, milk will appear to curdle.) Pour into a flat cake pan. Freeze. Break into pieces and process in a food processor or blender into a slush. Serve in disposable plastic V-shaped coffee-liner cups.

Yield: 6 servings
Exchange, 1 serving: negligible
Calories, 1 serving: 15
Carbohydrates, 1 serving: 1 g

Great Grape Blaster

1 pkg. (4-serving)	sugar-free grape gelatin	1 pkg. (4-serving)
1 c.	boiling water	250 mL
1 c.	cold purple grape juice	250 mL

Dissolve the grape gelatin in the boiling water. Allow to cool to lukewarm. Stir in cold grape juice. Pour into a flat cake pan. Freeze. Break into pieces and process in a food processor or blender into a slush. Serve in disposable plastic V-shaped coffee-liner cups.

Yield: 6 servings
Exchange, 1 serving: ⅓ fruit
Calories, 1 serving: 23
Carbohydrates, 1 serving: 6 g

Rum Mocha Ice Cream

½ gal.	vanilla ice cream	1064 g
9 oz.	semisweet chocolate, finely chopped	255 g
3 T.	instant coffee powder	45 mL
¼ c.	dark rum	60 mL

Soften the ice cream in the refrigerator until it can be whipped with an electric beater. Melt the semisweet chocolate in a double boiler over warm water, stirring occasionally. Allow to cool slightly. Dissolve the instant coffee in the rum. Transfer the ice cream to a large mixing bowl. Whip the ice cream on LOW, slowly pour the cooled melted chocolate into the ice cream, and continue beating until chocolate is completely incorporated. Gradually pour in coffee-rum mixture, and continue beating. Transfer ice cream to a covered freezer container. Freeze for several hours before serving. If ice cream becomes solid, allow to soften slightly in refrigerator before serving.

Yield: 16 servings
Exchange, 1 serving: 1 bread, 3 fat
Calories, 1 serving: 210
Carbohydrates, 1 serving: 16 g

Limey Lime Blaster

1 pkg. (4-serving)	sugar-free lime gelatin	1 pkg. (4-serving)
1 c.	boiling water	250 mL
1 c.	cold limeade	250 mL

Dissolve the lime gelatin in the boiling water. Allow to cool to lukewarm. Stir in cold limeade. Pour into a flat cake pan. Freeze. Break into pieces and process in a food processor or blender into a slush. Serve in disposable plastic V-shaped coffee-liner cups.

Yield: 6 servings
Exchange, 1 serving: negligible
Calories, 1 serving: 17
Carbohydrates, 1 serving: 5 g

Choco-sicles

1 pkg. (4-serving)	chocolate-flavored sugar-free instant pudding mix	1 pkg. (4-serving)
2¾ c.	skim milk	690 mL

Combine chocolate pudding mix and skim milk in a 1-qt. (1-L) measuring cup. Thoroughly blend with a wire whip or use an electric mixer and beat on SLOW for 3 to 4 minutes or until mixture is very smooth and begins to thicken. Pour into 10 popsicle forms. Freeze.

Yield: 10 servings
Exchange, 1 serving: ½ skim milk
Calories, 1 serving: 37
Carbohydrates, 1 serving: 6 g

White Chocolate Ice Cream with Fresh Peaches

½ gal.	vanilla ice cream	1064 g
8 oz.	white dietetic chocolate, chopped fine	227 g
2 jars	baby peaches	2 jars
(4-oz.)		(113-g)
2	fresh peaches	2

Soften the ice cream in the refrigerator until it can be whipped with an electric beater. Melt the white chocolate in a double boiler over warm water, stirring occasionally. Allow to cool slightly. Transfer the ice cream to a large mixing bowl. Whip the ice cream on LOW, slowly pour the cooled melted chocolate into the ice cream, and continue beating until chocolate is completely incorporated. Gradually pour in peach puree, and continue beating until smooth. Transfer ice cream to a covered freezer container. Freeze for several hours before serving. If ice cream becomes solid, allow to soften slightly in refrigerator before serving. Just before serving, peel, pit, and slice the peaches. Use sliced peaches as garnish.

Yield: 16 servings
Exchange, 1 serving: 1 bread, 2½ fat
Calories, 1 serving: 193
Carbohydrates, 1 serving: 15 g

Fresh Raspberry Ice Cream

½ gal.	vanilla ice cream	1064 g
1 qt.	fresh raspberries	1 L
1 T.	granulated fructose	15 mL

Soften the ice cream in the refrigerator until it can be whipped with an electric beater. Wash and clean the raspberries. Transfer to a medium-sized bowl. With a fork, slightly crush raspberries. Sprinkle with fructose. Stir, cover, and allow to rest 30 minutes. Transfer the ice cream to a large mixing bowl. Whip the ice cream on LOW until smooth. Fold in the crushed raspberries, allowing the raspberries to marbleize the ice cream. Transfer ice cream to a covered freezer container. Freeze for several hours before serving. If ice cream becomes solid, allow to soften slightly in refrigerator before serving.

Yield: 16 servings
Exchange, 1 serving: 1 bread, 1 fruit, 1 fat
Calories, 1 serving: 185
Carbohydrates, 1 serving: 28 g

Toasted Walnut and Chocolate Chip Ice Cream

½ gal.	vanilla ice cream	1064 g
1 c.	English walnut pieces	250 mL
½ c.	semisweet mini–chocolate chips	125 mL

Let the ice cream soften in the refrigerator until it can be whipped with an electric beater. Meanwhile, place walnuts in a nonstick frying pan. Place over medium-low heat, shaking pan occasionally to toast the walnuts. Remove from heat and allow to cool completely. Transfer the ice cream to a large mixing bowl. Whip the ice cream on LOW until smooth. Fold in the toasted walnuts and chocolate chips. Transfer ice cream to a covered freezer container. Freeze for several hours before serving. If ice cream becomes solid, allow to soften slightly in refrigerator before serving.

Yield: 16 servings
Exchange, 1 serving: 1 bread, 3 fat
Calories, 1 serving: 213
Carbohydrates, 1 serving: 17 g

Fresh Apple Cinnamon Ice Cream

2 T.	margarine	30 mL
3 large	red Delicious apples, peeled, cored, and chopped	3 large
2 in.	cinnamon stick	5 cm
½ gal.	vanilla ice cream	1064 g

Melt margarine in a heavy frying pan over medium heat. Add apples and cinnamon stick. Sauté for 5 minutes. Remove from heat and cool completely; discard cinnamon stick. Allow the ice cream to soften in the refrigerator until it can be whipped with an electric beater. Transfer the ice cream to a large mixing bowl. Whip the ice cream on LOW until smooth. Fold in the apple mixture. Transfer ice cream to a covered freezer container. Freeze for several hours before serving. If ice cream becomes solid, allow to soften slightly in refrigerator before serving.

Yield: 16 servings
Exchange, 1 serving: 1 bread, 1½ fat
Calories, 1 serving: 149
Carbohydrates, 1 serving: 16 g

Fillings, Frostings & Sauces

Fillings, frostings, and sauces are often neglected as an addition to a simple dessert. Yet, easy to make, they can do wonders in dressing up a dip of vanilla ice cream or a slice of plain white cake.

All fruits, fresh or frozen, become a filling or sauce simply by processing them in a food processor or blender. Since sauces are an opportunity to use frozen fruits, there is no need to make them up in advance. To add a little more interest and zip to your sauces, you can use any of the numerous flavorings that are now on the market. For instance, try blending a few sweet cherries with the addition of a small amount of brandy flavoring. Pour this over a slice of cake and your dessert will be beautiful and complete.

Try using the fillings as frosting, the frostings as filling, and the sauces instead of either one, for exciting new dessert treats. Use them for visual interest as well. Place the sauce under or alongside a slice of cake. Or spoon a small amount of frosting, filling, or sauce on top of a custard, pudding, or sliced fresh fruit. Then sprinkle a small amount of special topping on for added flavor, texture, and appeal. Colored cereals or stale cookies crushed to crumbs and nuts ground very fine make good toppings, and instant chocolate pudding can be used as a sauce.

Strawberry Filling

2 c.	frozen unsweetened strawberries	500 mL
2 T.	water	30 mL
4 t.	cornstarch	20 mL
2 T.	granulated sugar replacement	30 mL

Combine frozen strawberries, water, and cornstarch in a microwave bowl or saucepan. Cook in the microwave on HIGH for 3 to 4 minutes or until mixture is clear and thickened; stir at least once during cooking. Or, on top of the stove, cook in a saucepan on medium heat until mixture is clear and thickened. Remove from microwave or stove, and stir in sugar replacement. Allow to cool until mixture drops from a spoon in large blobs. Spread about two-thirds to three-fourths of the mixture between any number of cake layers. Reserve remaining filling for top decoration.

Yield: 8 servings
Exchange, 1 serving: ¼ fruit
Calories, 1 serving: 11
Carbohydrates, 1 serving: 3 g

Plain and Simple Prune Filling

| 1 c. | prunes | 250 mL |
| ½ t. | cinnamon | 2 mL |

Place prunes in a saucepan. Cover with water and simmer for 20 to 30 minutes until prunes are tender; then drain. Remove pits and mash with fork or process in food processor or blender. Stir in cinnamon.

Yield: 10 servings
Exchange, 1 serving: ⅓ fruit
Calories, 1 serving: 26
Carbohydrates, 1 serving: 7 g

Lemon Filling

2 T.	granulated fructose	30 mL
2 T.	cornstarch	30 mL
1¼ c.	evaporated skim milk	310 mL
3 T.	lemon juice	45 mL
1 T.	grated lemon rind	15 mL

Combine fructose and cornstarch in a heavy or nonstick saucepan. Blend in the milk and lemon juice. Cook and stir over medium heat until clear and thickened. Remove from heat and stir in the lemon rind. Cover and cool to room temperature, stirring occasionally.

Yield: 10 servings
Exchange, 1 serving: ½ bread
Calories, 1 serving: 34
Carbohydrates, 1 serving: 7 g

Almond Filling

5	egg whites	5
dash	salt	dash
2 T.	granulated fructose	30 mL
2 T.	granulated sugar replacement	30 mL
½ t.	ground cinnamon	2 mL
⅓ c.	ground almonds	90 mL

Combine egg whites and salt in a bowl. Beat until stiff. Gradually beat in the fructose and sugar replacement. Beat in cinnamon. Fold in the ground almonds. Refrigerate until ready to use.

Yield: 10 servings
Exchange, 1 serving: negligible
Calories, 1 serving: 9
Carbohydrates, 1 serving: 1 g

Chocolate Cream Filling

3 c.	skim milk	750 mL
¼ c.	carob powder	60 mL
¼ c.	granulated fructose	60 mL
6 T.	cornstarch	90 mL
½ t.	salt	2 mL
3	eggs, beaten	3
1 T.	margarine	15 mL
2 t.	vanilla extract	10 mL

Combine milk, carob powder, fructose, cornstarch, and salt in a heavy saucepan. Stir to dissolve cornstarch. Cook and stir over medium heat until thick. Cover, reduce heat, and cook 10 minutes longer. Stir a small amount of hot mixture into the beaten eggs. Return egg mixture to saucepan. Cook and stir for about 5 minutes. Remove from heat and stir in margarine until melted. Cover and allow to cool. Stir in vanilla before using.

Yield: 16 servings
Exchange, 1 serving: ⅔ bread, ½ fat
Calories, 1 serving: 63
Carbohydrates, 1 serving: 8 g

Vanilla Cream Filling

3 c.	skim milk	750 mL
¼ c.	granulated fructose	60 mL
6 T.	cornstarch	90 mL
½ t.	salt	2 mL
3	eggs, beaten	3
1 T.	margarine	15 mL
2 t.	vanilla extract	10 mL

Combine milk, fructose, cornstarch, and salt in a heavy saucepan. Stir to dissolve cornstarch. Cook and stir over medium heat until thick. Cover, reduce heat, and cook 10 minutes longer. Stir a small amount of hot mixture into the beaten eggs. Return egg mixture to saucepan. Cook and stir for about 5 minutes. Remove from heat and stir in margarine until melted. Cover and allow to cool. Stir in vanilla before using.

Yield: 16 servings
Exchange, 1 serving: ½ bread, ½ fat
Calories, 1 serving: 56
Carbohydrates, 1 serving: 6 g

Raspberry Filling

1 c.	fresh or frozen unsweetened raspberries	250 mL
2 T.	cornstarch	30 mL
1 T.	granulated sugar replacement	15 mL
¾ c.	evaporated skim milk	190 mL
2 t.	lemon juice	10 mL

Process ½ c. (125 mL) of the raspberries in a food processor or blender until pureed. Combine the cornstarch and sugar replacement in a heavy or nonstick saucepan; then gradually add the milk, pureed raspberries, and lemon juice. Cook and stir over medium heat until clear and thickened. Remove from heat and stir in remaining raspberries. Cover and cool to room temperature before using.

Yield: 10 servings
Exchange, 1 serving: ⅓ bread
Calories, 1 serving: 27
Carbohydrates, 1 serving: 5 g

Raisin Currant Filling

¼ c.	raisins	60 mL
¼ c.	currants	60 mL
¼ c.	cold water	60 mL
1 T.	all-purpose flour	15 mL
1 T.	lemon juice	15 mL
2 t.	grated lemon rind	10 mL

Combine all ingredients in a saucepan. Stir to dissolve flour. Cook over low heat until thick. Remove from heat, and allow to cool before using.

Yield: 10 servings
Exchange, 1 serving: ½ fruit
Calories, 1 serving: 24
Carbohydrates, 1 serving: 6 g

Spicy Mincemeat Filling

1 c.	raisins	250 mL
¼ c.	cider vinegar	60 mL
2 t.	cornstarch	10 mL
1 t.	ground cinnamon	5 mL
½ t.	ground nutmeg	2 mL
½ t.	ground allspice	2 mL
¼ t.	ground cloves	1 mL

Combine all ingredients in a saucepan. Stir to dissolve cornstarch. Cook and stir over low heat until thick. Remove from heat, and allow to cool before using.

Yield: 10 servings
Exchange, 1 serving: ⅔ fruit
Calories, 1 serving: 42
Carbohydrates, 1 serving: 11 g

Poppy Seed Filling

½ c.	water	125 mL
¼ c.	granulated fructose	60 mL
¼ c.	ground poppy seeds*	60 mL

⅓ c.	cold water	90 mL
1 T.	cornstarch	15 mL
½ t.	lemon juice	2 mL
¼ t.	ground cinnamon	1 mL
¼ t.	banana or butter rum flavoring	1 mL

*I use an electric coffee grinder to grind the poppy seeds, but they can be purchased ground in most Hungarian food stores.

Combine the ½ c. of water and the fructose in a small nonstick saucepan. Cook over medium heat, stirring until fructose is dissolved. Bring to a boil and boil for 3 minutes. Reduce heat and add ground poppy seeds. Dissolve cornstarch in the cold water. Add cornstarch solution, lemon juice, and cinnamon to poppy seed mixture. Cook and stir until mixture is thickened. Remove from heat, and stir in flavoring.

Yield: 10 servings
Exchange, 1 serving: ⅕ fruit
Calories, 1 serving: 13
Carbohydrates, 1 serving: 3 g

Chocolate Custard Frosting and Filling

2 c.	water	500 mL
3 T.	cornstarch	45 mL
2 T.	granulated fructose	30 mL
2 t.	vanilla extract	10 mL
1	egg yolk	1
4.5-oz. box	fructose-sweetened white frosting mix	128-g box
1 T.	water	15 mL
1 oz.	baking chocolate, melted	28 g

Combine water, cornstarch, fructose, vanilla extract, and egg yolk in a nonstick saucepan. Cook and stir over medium heat until mixture is very thick. Transfer to a large, preferably narrow, mixing bowl. Chill thoroughly. Beat slightly. Add frosting mix and 1 T. (15 mL) of water. Beat until thoroughly blended. Beat in melted chocolate, and continue beating until smooth and creamy for spreading.

Yield: 10 servings
Exchange, 1 serving: 1⅓ fruit, ½ fat
Calories, 1 serving: 89
Carbohydrates, 1 serving: 13 g

Custard Frosting and Filling

2 c.	water	500 mL
3 T.	cornstarch	45 mL
2 t.	vanilla extract	10 mL
1	egg yolk	1
4.5 oz. box	fructose-sweetened white frosting mix	128-g box
1 T.	any flavoring or extract	15 mL
	food coloring, if desired	

Combine water, cornstarch, vanilla extract, and egg yolk in a nonstick saucepan. Cook and stir over medium heat until mixture is very thick. Transfer to a large, preferably narrow, mixing bowl. Chill thoroughly. Beat in frosting mix and flavoring or extract of your choice. Add food coloring, if desired. Beat until smooth and creamy for spreading.

Yield: 10 servings
Exchange, 1 serving: 1⅓ fruit, ½ fat
Calories, 1 serving: 74
Carbohydrates, 1 serving: 13 g

Cappuccino Frosting

1 t.	unflavored gelatin	5 mL
2 T.	cold water	30 mL
3 T.	granulated fructose	45 mL
2 T.	instant coffee powder	30 mL
½ t.	ground cinnamon	2 mL
1 env.	nondairy whipped topping powder	1 env.
½ c.	skim milk	125 mL
1 t.	vanilla extract	5 mL

Sprinkle gelatin over cold water in a small saucepan. Allow to soften for 1 minute. Stir over low heat until gelatin is dissolved. Stir in fructose, instant coffee powder, and cinnamon. Stir until all ingredients are dissolved. Remove from heat and allow to cool to lukewarm. Combine nondairy topping powder and skim milk in a large, preferably narrow, bowl. Whip into soft peaks. Slowly beat in vanilla and lukewarm gelatin mixture. Beat to stiff peaks. Do not overbeat.

Yield: 20 servings
Exchange, 1 serving: ¼ bread
Calories, 1 serving: 21
Carbohydrates, 1 serving: 2 g

Maple Icing

2	egg whites	2
2 T.	Cary's Sugar-Free Maple-Flavored Syrup	30 mL
1 t.	maple flavoring	5 mL

Beat egg whites until stiff. Beating constantly, slowly pour maple syrup into egg whites. Beat in maple flavoring.

Yield: 10 servings
Exchange, 1 serving: negligible
Calories, 1 serving: 5
Carbohydrates, 1 serving: 1 g

Caramel-Flavored Frosting

1 box	butterscotch-flavored sugar-free	1 box
(4-serving)	to-cook pudding mix	(4-serving)
2 c.	water	500 mL
1	egg white	1

Combine butterscotch pudding mix and water in a saucepan. Cook and stir over medium heat until mixture comes to a full boil. Pour into mixing bowl and cool completely until set. Beat egg white until stiff. Beat egg white into cooled pudding just before using.

Yield: 10 servings
Exchange, 1 serving: negligible
Calories, 1 serving: 9
Carbohydrates, 1 serving: 1 g

Peanut Butter Frosting

⅔ c.	creamy peanut butter	180 mL
⅓ c.	granulated brown-sugar replacement	90 mL
¼ c.	skim milk	60 mL

Cream peanut butter with the brown-sugar replacement. Gradually beat in the milk. Beat to spreading consistency.

Yield: 10 servings
Exchange, 1 serving: ⅓ bread, 1½ fat
Calories, 1 serving: 97
Carbohydrates, 1 serving: 3 g

Seven-Minute Frosting

½ c.	granulated sugar replacement	125 mL
2	egg whites	2
½ t.	cream of tartar	2 mL
¼ c.	cold water	60 mL
2 t.	vanilla extract	10 mL

Simmer a small amount of water in the bottom of a double boiler. In the top of the boiler, combine sugar replacement, egg whites, cream of tartar, and the cold water. Set over the simmering water. Beat the egg white mixture on HIGH for 6 to 7 minutes or until very thick. Add the vanilla extract and beat a minute longer or until frosting is thick enough to spread.

Yield: 10 servings
Exchange, 1 serving: negligible
Calories, 1 serving: 3
Carbohydrates, 1 serving: 1 g

Peach Melba Frosting

1 t.	unflavored gelatin	5 mL
2 T.	cold water	30 mL
2 T.	granulated fructose	30 mL
1 env.	nondairy whipped topping powder	1 env.
½ c.	skim milk	125 mL
1 t.	vanilla extract	5 mL
3	fresh peaches, peeled and pureed	3
1 c.	fresh raspberries	250 mL

Sprinkle gelatin over cold water in a small saucepan. Allow to soften for 1 minute. Stir over low heat until gelatin is dissolved. Stir in fructose until dissolved. Remove from heat and allow to cool to lukewarm. Combine nondairy topping powder and skim milk in a large, preferably narrow, bowl. Whip into soft peaks. Slowly beat in vanilla, lukewarm gelatin mixture, and peach puree. Beat to stiff peaks. Fold in raspberries.

Yield: 20 servings
Exchange, 1 serving: ⅓ fruit
Calories, 1 serving: 30
Carbohydrates, 1 serving: 4 g

Semisweet Carob Frosting

¼ c.	carob powder	60 mL
2 T.	cornstarch	30 mL
1 T.	granulated fructose	15 mL
dash	salt	dash
½ c.	boiling water	125 mL
2 t.	vegetable oil	10 mL
1 t.	vanilla extract	5 mL

Combine carob powder, cornstarch, fructose, and salt in a small saucepan. Add boiling water. Stir to blend. Place over medium heat, and stir and cook until thick. Remove from heat. Stir in vegetable oil and vanilla thoroughly. Frost cake while frosting is still warm.

Yield: 10 servings
Exchange, 1 serving: ⅓ bread
Calories, 1 serving: 26
Carbohydrates, 1 serving: 4 g

Orange Frosting

1 c.	orange juice	250 mL
2 T.	cornstarch	30 mL
1 T.	granulated fructose	15 mL
dash	salt	dash
2 t.	vegetable oil	10 mL
1 t.	lemon extract	5 mL
½ t.	grated orange rind	2 mL

Combine orange juice, cornstarch, fructose, and salt in a small saucepan. Place over medium heat, and stir and cook until thick. Remove from heat. Stir in vegetable oil, lemon extract, and orange rind. Frost cake while frosting is still warm.

Yield: 10 servings
Exchange, 1 serving: ½ fruit
Calories, 1 serving: 27
Carbohydrates, 1 serving: 4 g

Milk-Chocolate Frosting

¼ c.	carob powder	60 mL
2 T.	cornstarch	30 mL
1 T.	granulated fructose	15 mL
dash	salt	dash
½ c.	hot low-fat milk	125 mL
1 t.	vanilla extract	5 mL

Combine carob powder, cornstarch, fructose, and salt in a small saucepan. Add hot milk. Place over medium heat, and stir and cook until thick. Remove from heat. Stir in vanilla. Frost cake while frosting is still warm.

Yield: 10 servings
Exchange, 1 serving: ⅓ bread
Calories, 1 serving: 23
Carbohydrates, 1 serving: 5 g

Burnt-Sugar Frosting

1 c.	water	250 mL
2 T.	cornstarch	30 mL
2 T.	granulated fructose	30 mL
2 t.	burnt sugar flavoring	10 mL
¼ c.	fructose-sweetened white frosting mix	60 mL

Combine water, cornstarch, and fructose in a saucepan. Stir to dissolve cornstarch. Cook and stir over medium heat until mixture is very thick, about 4 to 5 minutes. Remove from heat. Stir in flavoring. Allow to cool slightly. Beat in frosting mix.

Yield: 10 servings
Exchange, 1 serving: ½ fruit
Calories, 1 serving: 31
Carbohydrates, 1 serving: 7 g

Lemon Sauce

¼ c.	granulated sugar replacement	60 mL
¼ c.	granulated fructose	60 mL
2 T.	cornstarch	30 mL
1¼ c.	water	310 mL

| ¼ c. | lemon juice | 60 mL |
| 1 t. | grated lemon rind | 5 mL |

Combine sugar replacement, fructose, and cornstarch in a heavy or non-stick saucepan. Slowly blend in the water and lemon juice. Cook and stir over medium heat until clear and thickened. Remove from heat, cool to room temperature, and stir in the lemon rind. Store in refrigerator.

Yield: 10 servings
Exchange, 1 serving: ¼ fruit
Calories, 1 serving: 15
Carbohydrates, 1 serving: 4 g

Orange Sauce

¼ c.	granulated sugar replacement	60 mL
2 T.	cornstarch	30 mL
1½ c.	fresh or frozen orange juice	375 mL
1 t.	grated orange peel	5 mL

Combine sugar replacement and cornstarch in a heavy or nonstick saucepan. Slowly blend in the orange juice. Cook and stir over medium heat until clear and thickened. Remove from heat, cool to room temperature, and stir in the orange peel. Store in refrigerator.

Yield: 10 servings
Exchange, 1 serving: ¼ fruit
Calories, 1 serving: 21
Carbohydrates, 1 serving: 5 g

Caramel Sauce

1 box	butterscotch-flavored sugar-free	1 box
(4-serving)	to-cook pudding mix	(4-serving)
3 c.	water	750 mL

Combine pudding mix and water in a saucepan. Bring to a boil, stirring to dissolve. Boil 1 minute longer. Remove from heat. Serve hot or cold.

Yield: 10 servings
Exchange, 1 serving: negligible
Calories, 1 serving: 8
Carbohydrates, 1 serving: 1 g

Crushed Pineapple Sauce

¼ c.	unsweetened pineapple juice	60 mL
1 T.	cornstarch	15 mL
2 T.	granulated fructose	30 mL
20-oz. can	unsweetened crushed pineapple in juice	560-g can

Combine pineapple juice and cornstarch in a saucepan. Stir to dissolve cornstarch. Stir in fructose and canned crushed pineapple with its juice. Stir and cook over medium heat until the sauce is thickened.

Yield: 10 servings
Exchange, 1 serving: ½ fruit
Calories, 1 serving: 27
Carbohydrates, 1 serving: 7 g

Fast Apricot Sauce

1 c.	all-natural apricot preserves	250 mL
⅓ c.	water	90 mL
½ t.	lemon juice	2 mL
¼ t.	brandy flavoring	1 mL

Combine apricot preserves and water in a saucepan. Bring to a boil. Simmer for 1 minute. Remove from heat, and stir in lemon juice and brandy flavoring. Serve hot or cold.

Yield: 10 servings
Exchange, 1 serving: 1 fruit
Calories, 1 serving: 57
Carbohydrates, 1 serving: 13 g

Fresh Ginger Sauce

1½ c.	boiling water	375 mL
1 T.	grated fresh ginger	15 mL
¼ c.	granulated sugar replacement	60 mL
¼ c.	granulated fructose	60 mL
2 T.	cornstarch	30 mL
1 t.	lemon juice	5 mL

Combine boiling water and fresh ginger in a measuring cup or bowl. Cover and allow to cool to room temperature. Combine sugar replacement, fructose, and cornstarch in a heavy or nonstick saucepan. Slowly blend in the ginger water and lemon juice. Cook and stir over medium heat until clear and thickened. Store in refrigerator.

Yield: 10 servings
Exchange, 1 serving: ¼ fruit
Calories, 1 serving: 15
Carbohydrates, 1 serving: 4 g

Peach Sauce

| 29-oz. can | sliced peaches in juice | 822-g can |
| 1 t. | vanilla or almond extract | 5 mL |

Pour peaches with juice and extract into a food processor or blender. Process into a puree. Serve cold or warm.

Yield: 10 servings
Exchange, 1 serving: ⅓ fruit
Calories, 1 serving: 22
Carbohydrates, 1 serving: 6 g

Brandy Sauce

3	egg yolks	3
2 T.	granulated fructose	30 mL
1 T.	all-purpose flour	15 mL
1 c.	skim milk, hot	250 mL
2 T.	brandy	30 mL

Beat together the egg yolks and fructose in a heavy saucepan or microwave bowl until light and fluffy. Add the flour and beat well. Slowly add the hot milk. Place over medium heat or microwave on MEDIUM until boiling. Stir occasionally. On top of the stove, lower heat and cook for several minutes. From the microwave, cover with plastic wrap and allow to rest for 5 minutes. Just before serving, stir in brandy. This sauce is best served warm.

Yield: 10 servings
Exchange, 1 serving: ⅓ low-fat milk
Calories, 1 serving: 36
Carbohydrates, 1 serving: 3 g

Chocolate-Flavored Sauce

¼ c.	carob powder	60 mL
1 T.	granulated fructose	15 mL
1 T.	cornstarch	15 mL
½ c.	skim milk	125 mL
½ c.	evaporated skim milk	125 mL
1 t.	vanilla extract	5 mL

Combine carob powder, fructose, and cornstarch in a heavy or nonstick saucepan. Slowly add skim milk and evaporated skim milk. Blend well. Cook and stir over medium heat until mixture is thick and smooth. Remove from heat, and stir in vanilla. Cover and cool before serving.

For Chocolate Mocha Sauce: Add 2 t. (10 mL) of instant coffee powder to the fructose-cornstarch mixture.

Yield: 10 servings
Exchange, 1 serving: ⅓ bread
Calories, 1 serving: 30
Carbohydrates, 1 serving: 6 g

Chocolate Orange Sauce

¼ c.	carob powder	60 mL
1 T.	granulated fructose	15 mL
1 T.	cornstarch	15 mL
1 c.	skim milk	250 mL
2 T.	orange-flavored liqueur	30 mL
1 t.	grated orange peel	5 mL

Combine carob powder, fructose, and cornstarch in a heavy or nonstick saucepan. Slowly add skim milk and blend well. Cook and stir over medium heat until mixture is thick and smooth. Remove from heat, and stir in the orange-flavored liqueur and orange peel. Cover and cool before serving.

Yield: 10 servings
Exchange, 1 serving: ⅓ skim milk
Calories, 1 serving: 25
Carbohydrates, 1 serving: 5 g

From the Kitchen of...

The recipes that follow are reprinted with permission of Bernard Food Industries, Inc.; Del Monte Foods; and Featherweight.

From the Kitchen of Bernard

No-Roll Pie Crust

1 box   Sweet 'n Low brand white cake mix
3 T.   water

Mix cake mix and water in mixer until batter is smooth, about 3 minutes. Lightly grease or spray with nonfat vegetable oil, coating bottom and sides of two 9-in. round pie pans. With a rubber spatula, spread batter to coat bottom and sides of the two pans. Bake at 350 °F for 12 to 15 minutes for recipes calling for prebaked pie shell, or fill with fruit and bake with filling.

Sufficient crust for 16 servings (eight cuts per 9-in. pie). Each serving of unfilled crust: 56 calories.

The second pie shell may be frozen for later use. Or batter not needed for a second pie may be baked as cookies (see white-cake-mix label for baking directions).

No-Roll Chocolate Pie Crust

1 box   Sweet 'n Low brand chocolate cake mix
3 T.   water

Follow directions for "No-Roll Pie Crust" (made with white cake mix).

Makes two 9-in. crusts, or one 9-in. crust and two-and-a-half dozen 1½-in.-diameter cookies.

Fill baked chocolate pie crust with low-calorie vanilla or chocolate pudding; garnish with low-calorie whipped topping. Use low-calorie product labels as a guide to calculate the caloric value of the finished pie.

Strawberry Bavarian Creme Pie

1	baked 9-in. "No-Roll Pie Crust"
1 qt. (1 lb.)	fresh or frozen unsweetened strawberries
½ t.	Sweet 'n Low granulated sugar substitute (sweetness of 2 T. of sugar)
1 c.	low-calorie whipped topping, whipped

See recipe for "No-Roll Pie Crust." Bake and cool crust. Sprinkle sugar substitute on fresh or frozen strawberries. Gently toss to distribute sweetener. Fold all but 1 c. of fruit into whipped topping and fill crust. Garnish with remaining fruit. If frozen strawberries are used, refrigerate pie until strawberries are slightly thawed. Loosen crust around rim before slicing.

Makes one 9-in. pie—eight servings—95 calories per serving.

Dutch Apple Pie

Crust

| ½ box (1 c.) | Sweet 'n Low brand white cake mix |
| 2 T. | water |

Filling

¼ t.	cinnamon
2 t.	Sweet 'n Low granulated sugar substitute (sweetness of ½ c. of sugar)
4 c.	sliced apples (4–5 apples), peeled and cored
½ c.	water

Topping

½ box (1 c.)	Sweet 'n Low brand white cake mix
¼ t.	cinnamon
¼ c.	low-fat cottage cheese (unsalted for sodium-restricted diets)

For crust: Mix 1 c. of cake mix with 2 T. of water. Lightly grease or spray with nonfat vegetable oil, coating bottom and sides of a 9-in. pie pan. With a rubber spatula, spread batter to coat bottom and sides of pan.

For filling: Mix ¼ t. of cinnamon with 2 t. of sugar substitute. Sprinkle on apples and toss until cinnamon and sweetener are well distributed. Place apple mixture in unbaked crust. Sprinkle apples with ½ c. of water.

For topping: Mix remaining cake mix and ¼ t. of cinnamon. Stir in cottage cheese and mix until crumbly. Sprinkle on top of apple filling.

Cover pie loosely with aluminum foil. Bake at 400 °F for 30 minutes; remove foil and bake until brown, approximately 15 minutes.

Makes one 9-in. pie—eight servings—163 calories per serving.

Chocolate Mint Cake

1 box	Sweet 'n Low brand chocolate cake mix
¼ t.	salt (omit if sodium-restricted)
½ t.	mint extract
⅔ c.	water

Mix cake mix, salt, mint extract, and half the water for 3 minutes in mixer. Add the balance of water and mix 1 minute. Pour batter into lightly greased and wax paper–lined 8-in. round or square pan. Bake at 375 °F for 25 minutes. Cool slightly before removing from pan.

Makes one 8-in. single-layer cake—10 servings—90 calories per serving. If frosted with ⅓ c. of Sweet 'n Low brand white frosting, each serving would be 120 calories.

Or, drizzle cake with 2 T. of "Chocolate Fudge Topping" (see recipe on page 343), to which may be added a drop of mint extract. One serving of cake with drizzled topping would be 108 calories.

Spice Cake

1 box	Sweet 'n Low brand white cake mix
½ t.	cinnamon
¼ t.	salt (omit if sodium-restricted)
⅛ t.	cloves
⅔ c.	water

Combine cake mix and spices in mixing bowl. Add half the water and mix 3 minutes in mixer. Add the balance of water and mix 1 minute. Pour batter into lightly greased and wax paper–lined 8-in. baking pan. Bake at 375 °F for 25 minutes. Cool slightly before removing from pan.

Makes 10 servings—90 calories per serving.

Peach Upside-Down Cake

1 lb.	can sliced peaches, juice pack
	(no sugar added)
1 box	Sweet 'n Low brand lemon cake mix

Drain sliced peaches, reserving juice. Arrange peach slices in lightly greased and wax paper–lined 8-in. round pan. Mix cake mix with ⅓ c. of drained juice for 3 minutes in mixer. Add ⅓ c. of more juice and mix 1 minute. Pour batter over peach slices. Bake at 375 °F for 30 to 40 minutes. Cool slightly. Loosen cake around the sides. Invert onto serving plate. Remove wax paper.

   Makes one 8-in. cake—110 calories per serving.

Chocolate-Fudge Topping

1 box	Sweet 'n Low brand white frosting mix
2½ T.	cocoa (unsweetened)
¼ c.	water

Mix frosting mix and cocoa in a saucepan. Stir in water. Bring to a boil while stirring. Makes 7 oz. of hot fudge topping. Drizzle from the tip of a · spoon over cake or low-calorie, low-cholesterol "ice cream."

   2 T. sufficient for an 8-in. layer—180 calories (or 18 calories per serving).

   1 T. sufficient for an 8 × 4 in. loaf—90 calories (or 9 calories per serving).

   1 t. sufficient for a scoop of "ice cream" or a cupcake—30 calories per teaspoon.

   Leftover fudge topping can be refrigerated if stored in a closed container. It will thicken when chilled. Leave at room temperature before using again, and then thin with a little water to desired consistency.

Lemon Frosting

1 box	Sweet 'n Low brand white frosting mix
¼ c.	hot water
4 t.	lemon juice
1 t.	lemon extract
3 drops	yellow food color

Empty frosting mix into a mixing bowl. Add water, lemon juice, lemon extract, and yellow food color. Beat until smooth and fluffy. Makes 1⅓ c. of frosting—to frost four 8-in. layers of cake (⅓ c. of frosting per layer).

   ⅓ c. of frosting equals 304 calories (30 calories per serving). 1½ t. of frosting (for one cupcake) equals 30 calories.

   Leftover frosting can be refrigerated if stored in a closed container.

From the Kitchen of Del Monte

Peach-Pear Tart

1 can (16-oz.)	Del Monte Lite Pear Halves
1 can (16-oz.)	Del Monte Lite Sliced Peaches
8 oz.	Neufchatel cheese or low-fat cream cheese, softened
1 t.	lemon juice
½ t.	grated lemon peel
1 (9-in.)	pastry shell, baked
⅓ c.	sliced almonds, toasted
2 T.	orange marmalade, melted

Drain fruit, reserving liquid. Boil liquid gently 20 minutes; cool. Combine cheese with 2 T. of the reduced liquid, the lemon juice, and the lemon peel. Beat until light. Spread cheese mixture over bottom of pastry shell. Sprinkle nuts over cheese mixture. Arrange fruit in alternate pattern on top. Brush with orange marmalade.* Garnish with additional almonds, if desired.

*You can thin orange marmalade with 1 t. of reduced liquid over low heat.

Calico Pears

1 can (16-oz.)	Del Monte Lite Pear Halves
1 T.	butter
⅓ c.	chopped cooked ham
½ c.	chopped onion
½ c.	chopped green pepper
¼ c.	grated Parmesan cheese
	chopped walnuts

Drain fruit, reserving liquid for other recipe uses. Place pears in baking dish; set aside. In skillet, heat butter. Lightly sauté ham, onion, green pepper, and Parmesan cheese. Top pears with ham mixture; sprinkle with nuts. Broil 3 to 5 minutes.

Yield: 3 to 4 servings

Lite Melon Meringue

2	small honeydews or cantaloupes
4	egg whites
2 t.	sugar
2 c.	plain yogurt or ice milk
1 can	Del Monte Lite Sliced Peaches
(16-oz.)	or Sliced Pears, drained

Cut melons in half. Seed. Whip egg whites with sugar until stiff. Fill melon halves with yogurt and place peach slices on top edge in pinwheel fashion. Top with meringue. Bake at 450 °F for 2 to 3 minutes or until lightly browned.

Yield: 4 servings

From the Kitchen of Featherweight

Raisin Cottage Delight

1 c.	low-fat cottage cheese
8	slices bread, toasted
4 t.	butter or margarine
4 T.	Featherweight red raspberry preserves
¼ c.	dark seedless raisins
	ground cinnamon

Purée cottage cheese. Spread each slice of toast with ½ t. of butter and 2 T. of cottage cheese. Spread ½ T. of preserves over cottage cheese. Sprinkle top with raisins and cinnamon.

Yield: 4 servings
Exchange, 1 serving: 1 fruit, 1 meat, 2 bread, 1 fat
Calories, 1 serving: 270

Minted Fruit

2	cans Featherweight juice pack
(16-oz.)	
	fruits for salad, drained
6 drops	Featherweight sweetening
12	Featherweight peppermint sugarless
	mini-mints

Combine fruit with sweetening in a bowl. Chill thoroughly. Crush mints between two spoons. Spoon chilled fruit into dessert dishes and sprinkle with crushed mints.

Yield: 6 servings
Exchange, 1 serving: 1 fruit
Calories: 73

Raspberry Parfait

½ pkg.	Featherweight raspberry gelatin
(1 env.)	(or any other flavor)
1 c.	boiling water
1 c.	cold water
1 env.	Featherweight whipped topping

Empty envelope of gelatin into bowl. Add boiling water and stir until dissolved. Add cold water and stir well. Chill until slightly thickened. Prepare whipped topping as directed on package. Blend ¾ c. of whipped topping into slightly thickened gelatin. Spoon half of gelatin mixture into parfait glasses. Chill until slightly thickened. Spoon half of remaining whipped topping on gelatin. Spoon remaining gelatin mixture over whipped topping. Chill until set. Top each parfait with a dollop of remaining whipped topping.

Yield: 4 servings
Exchange, 1 serving: free
Calories, 1 serving: 29

Hot Mocha Drink

1½ c.	skim milk
2 c.	strong coffee
½ pkg.	Featherweight chocolate pudding mix
(1 env.)	

Pour skim milk and coffee in a small saucepan; stir in pudding mix. Stir over low heat until mixture comes to a boil. Pour into mugs to serve.

Yield: 6 servings
Exchange, 1 serving: ½ milk
Calories, 1 serving: 31

Dessert Products Information

Food manufacturers now include nutritional information on the labels of their products. This information can be very useful to anyone using the American Diabetes Association's Exchange Lists in their diets. The labels show the number of calories and the grams of protein, carbohydrates, and fat in each serving. Most of the labels resemble the example that follows.

NUTRITIONAL INFORMATION PER SERVING
Servings per container: 12
Serving size (Cookie): 3
Calories per serving: 170
Protein: 2 g
Carbohydrates: 22 g
Fat: 7 g

With this information, you can work out the food exchange on any product. The following exchange list is needed for calculations.

Exchange	Calories	Carbohydrates (grams)	Protein (grams)	Fat (grams)
Starch/Bread	80	15	3	trace
Meat				
Lean	55	0	7	3
Medium-fat	75	0	7	5
High-fat	100	0	7	8
Vegetable	25	5	2	0
Fruit	60	15	0	0
Milk				
Skim	90	12	8	trace
Low-fat	120	12	8	5
Whole	150	12	8	8
Fat	45	0	0	5

Compare the nutrient value on the label with the nutrient value on the exchange list. Count whole and nearest half exchanges.

	Exchange	C	P	F
1. List the grams of carbohydrates, protein, and fat per serving.		22	2	7
2. Subtract carbohydrates first. Bread exchange has 15 g carbohydrates + 3 g protein.	1 bread	−15	−3	
		7	−1	7
3. Think about the ingredients in a cookie and compare the next-nearest carbohydrate exchange. Fruit has 15 g; ½ fruit has 7.5 or 7.	½ fruit	−7		
		0	−1	7
4. Compare the fat exchange.	1 fat			−5
			−1	2

You have 2 grams of fat left, or approximately ½ fat exchange; therefore, your exchange on 1 serving of this product is equivalent to 1 bread, ½ fruit, and 1½ fat.

5. Check with calories

   1 bread = 80 calories
   ½ fruit = 30 calories
   1½ fat = 67 calories

   Total: 177 calories (Product Information states 170)

It's important to realize that most exchanges figured on foods will vary because the averages are used for calculating the original exchange value.

Product Lists

The product lists that follow are reprinted with permission of Borden, Inc.; Campbell Soup Company; The Dannon Company, Inc.; Del Monte Foods; Featherweight; Flavorland Foods; Health Valley Foods; and Pepperidge Farm.

Remember these are only general reference lists. Many of the products' ingredients vary from area to area, and from season to season. You need to check the products' labels for the most recently updated information.

Borden Products

BORDEN FAT-FREE FROZEN DESSERTS

Vanilla
Serving size: ½ cup (4 oz.)
Servings per container: 16
Calories: 90
Protein: 3 g
Carbohydrates: 20 g
Fat: Less than 1 g

Chocolate
Serving size: ½ cup (4 oz.)
Servings per container: 16
Calories: 100
Protein: 3 g
Carbohydrates: 21 g
Fat: Less than 1 g

Strawberry
Serving size: ½ cup (4 oz.)
Servings per container: 16
Calories: 90
Protein: 3 g
Carbohydrates: 21 g
Fat: Less than 1 g

Peach
Serving size: ½ cup (4 oz.)
Servings per container: 16
Calories: 90
Protein: 2 g
Carbohydrates: 21 g
Fat: Less than 1 g

Black Cherry
Serving size: ½ cup (4 oz.)
Servings per container: 16
Calories: 90
Protein: 2 g
Carbohydrates: 21 g
Fat: Less than 1 g

OTHER BORDEN PRODUCTS

Vanilla-Flavored Ice Milk
Serving size: ½ cup (4 oz.)
Calories: 90
Protein: 2 g
Carbohydrates: 17 g
Fat: 2 g

Strawberry Ice Milk
Serving size: ½ cup (4 oz.)
Calories: 90
Protein: 2 g
Carbohydrates: 17 g
Fat: 2 g

Orange Sherbet
Serving size: ½ cup (4 oz.)
Calories: 110
Protein: 1 g
Carbohydrates: 25 g
Fat: 1 g

Cary's Sugar-Free
Maple-Flavored Syrup
Serving size: 1 tablespoon (15.5 g)
Servings per container: 25
Calories: 10
Protein: 0 g
Carbohydrates: 2 g
Fat: 0 g

Lite-Line Low-fat Cottage Cheese
(1½% milk fat)
Serving size: ½ cup (4 oz.)
Calories: 90
Protein: 14 g
Carbohydrates: 4 g
Fat: 2 g

Dry-Curd Cottage Cheese
(0.5% milk fat)
Serving size: ½ cup (4 oz.)
Calories: 80
Protein: 18 g
Carbohydrates: 3 g
Fat: 1 g

Campbell Soup Products

CAMPBELL'S JUICES

Juice Bowl, Apple
Serving size: 6 oz.
Calories: 110
Protein: 0 g
Carbohydrates: 25 g
Fat: 0 g

Juice Bowl, Grape
Serving size: 6 oz.
Calories: 110
Protein: 0 g
Carbohydrates: 27 g
Fat: 0 g

Juice Bowl, Grapefruit
Serving size: 6 oz.
Calories: 80
Protein: 0 g
Carbohydrates: 17 g
Fat: 0 g

Juice Bowl, Orange
Serving size: 6 oz.
Calories: 90
Protein: 0 g
Carbohydrates: 21 g
Fat: 0 g

Dannon Products

Plain Nonfat Yogurt
Serving size: 1 cup (8 oz.)
Calories: 110
Fat: 0 g

Plain Low-Fat Yogurt
Serving size: 1 cup (8 oz.)
Calories: 140
Fat: 4 g

Lemon (or Vanilla) Low-Fat Yogurt
Serving size: 1 cup (8 oz.)
Calories: 200
Fat: 3 g

Del Monte Products

FRUIT NATURALS

Sliced Yellow Cling Peaches in Peach Juice
Serving size: ½ c. (4 oz.)
Calories: 60
Protein: 0 g
Carbohydrates: 15 g
Fat: 0 g

Bartlett Pear Halves in Pear Juice
Serving size: ½ c. (4 oz.)
Calories: 60
Protein: 0 g
Carbohydrates: 16 g
Fat: 0 g

Fruit Cocktail in Juices
Serving size: ½ c. (4 oz.)
Calories: 60
Protein: 0 g
Carbohydrates: 15 g
Fat: 0 g

Chunky Mixed Fruit in Juices
Serving size: ½ c. (4 oz.)
Calories: 50
Protein: 0 g
Carbohydrates: 14 g
Fat: 0 g

Featherweight Products

LOW-CALORIE FRUIT SPREADS

For Strawberry, Grape, Apple, and Blackberry Jelly, and for Apricot, Blackberry, Peach, Red Raspberry, and Strawberry Preserves:
Serving size: 1 t
Calories: 4
Protein: 0 g
Carbohydrates: 1 g
Fat: 0 g

LOW-CALORIE SYRUPS

For Blueberry and Pancake Syrups:
Serving size: 1 T
Calories: 16
Protein: 0 g
Carbohydrates: 4 g
Fat: 0 g

SWEETENERS

Liquid Sweetening
Serving size: 3 dps.
Calories: 0
Protein: 0 g
Carbohydrates: 0 g
Fat: 0 g

Fructose Sweetener
Serving size: 1 t
Calories: 12
Protein: 0 g
Carbohydrates: 3 g
Fat: 0 g

FRUIT

JP Apricot Halves
Serving size: ½ c
Calories: 50
Protein: 1 g
Carbohydrates: 12 g
Fat: 0 g

JP Fruit Cocktail
Serving size: ½ c
Calories: 50
Protein: 1 g
Carbohydrates: 14 g
Fat: 0 g

JP Yellow Cling Peach Halves, Slices
Serving size: ½ c
Calories: 50
Protein: 0 g
Carbohydrates: 14 g
Fat: 0 g

WP Mandarin Oranges
Serving size: ½ c
Calories: 35
Protein: 0 g
Carbohydrates: 8 g
Fat: 0 g

JP Pear Halves
Serving size: ½ c
Calories: 60
Protein: 0 g
Carbohydrates: 15 g
Fat: 0 g

JP Pineapple Slices
Serving size: ½ c
Calories: 70
Protein: 0 g
Carbohydrates: 18 g
Fat: 0 g

WP Applesauce
Serving size: ½ c
Calories: 50
Protein: 0 g
Carbohydrates: 12 g
Fat: 0 g

JP Fruit Salad
Serving size: ½ c
Calories: 50
Protein: 1 g
Carbohydrates: 13 g
Fat: 0 g

JP Grapefruit Segments
Serving size: ½ c
Calories: 40
Protein: 0 g
Carbohydrates: 9 g
Fat: 0 g

LOW-SODIUM/LOW-CALORIE NUTRASWEET DESSERTS

For Butterscotch, Chocolate, and Vanilla Puddings:
Serving size: ½ c
Calories: 12
Protein: 0 g
Carbohydrates: 3 g
Fat: 0 g

For Raspberry, Strawberry, Cherry, Lemon, Lime, and Orange Gelatins:
Serving size: ½ c
Calories: 10
Protein: 2 g
Carbohydrates: 1 g
Fat: 0 g

For Vanilla and Butterscotch Instant Puddings:
Serving size: ½ c
Calories: 100
Protein: 4 g
Carbohydrates: 19 g
Fat: 0 g

For Vanilla and Lemon Custards:
Serving size: ½ c
Calories: 40
Protein: 1 g
Carbohydrates: 8 g
Fat: 0 g

CANDY

For Milk Chocolate and Chocolate Crunch Bars:
Serving size: 1 section
Calories: 80
Protein: 1 g
Carbohydrates: 7 g
Fat: 6 g

Caramels
Serving size: 1 piece
Calories: 30
Protein: 0 g
Carbohydrates: 5 g
Fat: 1 g

COOKIES

For Chocolate Chip, Double Chocolate Chip, Lemon, Vanilla, and Oatmeal Raisin Cookies:
Serving size: 1 cookie
Calories: 45
Protein: 1 g
Carbohydrates: 6 g
Fat: 2 g

For Chocolate, Vanilla, and Strawberry Creme Wafers:
Serving size: 1 wafer
Calories: 20
Protein: 0 g
Carbohydrates: 3 g
Fat: 1 g

Flavorland Products

FROZEN FRUITS

Blackberries
Serving size: 4 oz.
Servings per package: 4
Calories: 70
Protein: 1 g
Carbohydrates: 18 g
Fat: 0 g

Black Raspberries
Serving size: 4 oz.
Servings per package: 3
Calories: 60
Protein: 1 g
Carbohydrates: 13 g
Fat: 1 g

Blueberries
Serving size: 4 oz.
Servings per package: 4
Calories: 60
Protein: 0 g
Carbohydrates: 14 g
Fat: 1 g

Boysenberries
Serving size: 4 oz.
Servings per package: 4
Calories: 60
Protein: 1 g
Carbohydrates: 14 g
Fat: 0 g

Melon Balls
Serving size: 4 oz.
Servings per package: 4
Calories: 35
Protein: 1 g
Carbohydrates: 9 g
Fat: 0 g

Peach Slices
Serving size: 4 oz.
Servings per package: 4
Calories: 50
Protein: 1 g
Carbohydrates: 13 g
Fat: 0 g

Red Raspberries
Serving size: 4 oz.
Servings per package: 3
Calories: 60
Protein: 2 g
Carbohydrates: 13 g
Fat: 0 g

Rhubarb
Serving size: 4 oz.
Servings per package: 4
Calories: 25
Protein: 1 g
Carbohydrates: 6 g
Fat: 0 g

Deluxe Fruit Mix
Serving size: 4 oz.
Servings per package: 4
Calories: 50
Protein: 1 g
Carbohydrates: 13 g
Fat: 0 g

Dark Sweet Cherries
Serving size: 4 oz.
Servings per package: 4
Calories: 80
Protein: 1 g
Carbohydrates: 19 g
Fat: 1 g

Fruit Medley
Serving size: 4 oz.
Servings per package: 4
Calories: 60
Protein: 1 g
Carbohydrates: 14 g
Fat: 1 g

Red Tart Cherries
Serving size: 4 oz.
Servings per package: 4
Calories: 50
Protein: 1 g
Carbohydrates: 12 g
Fat: 0 g

Whole Strawberries
Serving size: 4 oz.
Servings per package: 4
Calories: 40
Protein: 0 g
Carbohydrates: 10 g
Fat: 0 g

Health Valley Products

COOKIES

For Fancy Fruit Chunks—Apricot Almond, Date Pecan, and Tropical Fruit:
Serving size: 2 cookies
Calories: 90
Exchanges: ½ starch
      ½ fruit
      ½ fat

For Fat-Free Cookies—Apple Spice, Apricot Delight, Date Delight, Hawaiian Fruit, and Raisin Oatmeal:
Serving size: 3 cookies
Calories: 75
Exchanges: ½ starch
      ½ fruit

For Fruit Jumbos—Almond Date, Raisin Nut, Oat Bran, and Tropical Fruit; and for Honey Jumbos— Crisp Cinnamon and Crisp Peanut Butter:
Serving size: 1 cookie
Calories: 70
Exchanges: 1 starch

The Great Tofu Cookie
Serving size: 2 cookies
Calories: 90
Exchanges: ½ starch
      ½ fruit
      ½ fat

The Great Wheat-Free Cookie
Serving size: 2 cookies
Calories: 130
Exchanges: ½ starch
           ½ fruit
           ½ fat

SNACK BARS

For 100% Organic Fat-Free Fruit Bars—Apple, Apricot, Date, and Raisin:
Serving size: 1 bar
Calories: 140
Exchanges: 1 starch
           1 fruit

For Oat Bran Jumbo Fruit Bars—Almond & Date and Fruit & Nut:
Serving size: 1 bar
Calories: 170
Exchanges: 1 starch
           ½ fruit
           1 fat

Pepperidge Farm Products

FROZEN PRODUCTS

Puff Pastry Sheets
Serving size: ¼ sheet
Calories: 260
Protein: 4 g
Carbohydrates: 22 g
Fat: 17 g

Puff Pastry Shells
Serving size: 1
Calories: 210
Protein: 2 g
Carbohydrates: 17 g
Fat: 15 g

COOKIES

Bordeaux
Serving size: 2 cookies
Calories: 70
Protein: 1 g
Carbohydrates: 11 g
Fat: 3 g

Chantilly
Serving size: 1 cookie
Calories: 80
Protein: 1 g
Carbohydrates: 14 g
Fat: 2 g

Zurich
Serving size: 1 cookie
Calories: 60
Protein: 1 g
Carbohydrates: 10 g
Fat: 2 g

Ginger Man
Serving size: 2 cookies
Calories: 70
Protein: 1 g
Carbohydrates: 10 g
Fat: 3 g

Molasses Crisp
Serving size: 2 cookies
Calories: 70
Protein: 1 g
Carbohydrates: 8 g
Fat: 3 g

Apricot Raspberry/Strawberry
Serving size: 2 cookies
Calories: 100
Protein: 1 g
Carbohydrates: 15 g
Fat: 4 g (strawberry: 5 g)

Orleans
Serving size: 3 cookies
Calories: 90
Protein: 0 g
Carbohydrates: 11 g
Fat: 6 g

CAKES

Cherry Cake Supreme
Serving size: 3¼ oz.
Calories: 170
Protein: 0 g
Carbohydrates: 38 g
Fat: 2 g
Diet exchange: 1 starch
              1 fruit
              ½ fat

Lemon Cake Supreme
Serving size: 2¼ oz.
Calories: 170
Protein: 4 g
Carbohydrates: 26 g
Fat: 5 g
Diet exchange: 1½ starch
              1 fat

Raspberry Vanilla Swirl
Serving size: 3¼ oz.
Calories: 160
Protein: 4 g
Carbohydrates: 25 g
Fat: 5 g
Diet exchange: 1 starch
              ½ fruit
              1 fat

Chocolate Mousse Cake
Serving size: 2½ oz.
Calories: 190
Protein: 3 g
Carbohydrates: 25 g
Fat: 9 g
Diet exchange: 1½ starch
              2 fat

Strawberry Shortcake
Serving size: 3 oz.
Calories: 170
Protein: 2 g
Carbohydrates: 30 g
Fat: 5 g
Diet exchange: 1½ starch
              1 fat

Apple 'n Spice Bake
Serving size: 4¼ oz.
Calories: 170
Protein: 2 g
Carbohydrates: 37 g
Fat: 2 g
Diet exchange: 1 starch
              1 fruit
              ½ fat

EXCHANGE LISTS

The reason for dividing food into six different groups is that foods vary in their carbohydrate, protein, fat, and calorie content. Each exchange list contains foods that are alike – each choice contains about the same amount of carbohydrate, protein, fat, and calories.

The following chart shows the amount of these nutrients in one serving from each exchange list.

Exchange List	Carbohydrate (grams)	Protein (grams)	Fat (grams)	Calories
Starch/Bread	15	3	trace	80
Meat				
Lean	–	7	3	55
Medium-Fat	–	7	5	75
High-Fat	–	7	8	100
Vegetable	5	2	–	25
Fruit	15	–	–	60
Milk				
Skim	12	8	trace	90
Lowfat	12	8	5	120
Whole	12	8	8	150
Fat	–	–	5	45

As you read the exchange lists, you will notice that one choice often is a larger amount of food than another choice from the same list. Because foods are so different, each food is measured or weighed so the amount of carbohydrate, protein, fat, and calories is the same in each choice.

You will notice symbols on some foods in the exchange groups. Foods that are high in fiber (3 grams or more per exchange) have this 🌾 symbol. High-fiber foods are good for you. It is important to eat more of these foods.

Foods that are high in sodium (400 milligrams or more of sodium per exchange) have this 🦞 symbol; foods that have 400 mg or more of sodium if two or more exchanges are eaten have this ★ symbol. It's a good idea to limit your intake of high-salt foods, especially if you have high blood pressure.

If you have a favorite food that is not included in any of these groups, ask your dietitian about it. That food can probably be worked into your meal plan, at least now and then.

1
STARCH/BREAD LIST

Each item in this list contains approximately 15 grams of carbohydrate, 3 grams of protein, a trace of fat, and 80 calories. Whole grain products average about 2 grams of fiber per exchange. Some foods are higher in fiber. Those foods that contain 3 or more grams of fiber per exchange are identified with the fiber symbol 🌾.

You can choose your starch exchanges from any of the items on this list. If you want to eat a starch food that is not on this list, the general rule is that:

- 1/2 cup of cereal, grain or pasta is one exchange
- 1 ounce of a bread product is one exchange

Your dietitian can help you be more exact.

CEREALS/GRAINS/PASTA

🌾 Bran cereals, concentrated (such as Bran Buds® All Bran®)	1/3 cup
🌾 Bran cereals, flaked	1/2 cup
Bulgur (cooked)	1/2 cup
Cooked cereals	1/2 cup
Cornmeal (dry)	2 1/2 Tbsp.
Grape-Nuts®	3 Tbsp.
Grits (cooked)	1/2 cup
Other ready-to-eat unsweetened cereals	3/4 cup
Pasta (cooked)	1/2 cup
Puffed cereal	1 1/2 cup
Rice, white or brown (cooked)	1/3 cup
Shredded wheat	1/2 cup
🌾 Wheat germ	3 Tbsp.

DRIED BEANS/PEAS/LENTILS

🌾 Beans and peas (cooked) (such as kidney, white, split, blackeye)	1/3 cup
🌾 Lentils (cooked)	1/3 cup
🌾 Baked beans	1/4 cup

STARCHY VEGETABLES

🌾 Corn	1/2 cup
🌾 Corn on cob, 6 in. long	1
🌾 Lima beans	1/2 cup

🌾 Peas, green (canned or frozen)	1/2 cup
🌾 Plantain	1/2 cup
Potato, baked	1 small (3 oz.)
Potato, mashed	1/2 cup
🌾 Squash, winter (acorn, butternut)	1 cup
Yam, sweet potato, plain	1/3 cup

BREAD

Bagel	1/2 (1 oz.)
Bread sticks, crisp, 4 in. long × 1/2 in.	2 (2/3 oz.)
Croutons, lowfat	1 cup
English muffin	1/2
Frankfurter or hamburger bun	1/2 (1 oz.)
Pita, 6 in. across	1/2
Plain roll, small	1 (1 oz.)
Raisin, unfrosted	1 slice (1 oz.)
Rye, pumpernickel	1 slice (1 oz.)
Tortilla, 6 in. across	1
White (including French, Italian)	1 slice (1 oz.)
Whole wheat	1 slice (1 oz.)

🌾 3 grams or more of fiber per exchange

CRACKERS/SNACKS

Animal crackers	8
Graham crackers, 2 1/2 in. square	3
Matzoh	3/4 oz.
Melba toast	5 slices
Oyster crackers	24
Popcorn (popped, no fat added)	3 cups
Pretzels	3/4 oz.
🌾 Rye crisp, 2 in. × 3 1/2 in.	4
Saltine-type crackers	6
🌾 Whole-wheat crackers, no fat added (crisp breads, such as Finn®, Kavli®, Wasa®)	2-4 slices (3/4 oz.)
Taco shell, 6 in. across	2
Waffle, 4 1/2 in. square	1
🌾 Whole-wheat crackers, fat added (such as Triscuit®)	4-6 (1 oz.)

STARCH FOODS PREPARED WITH FAT

(Count as 1 starch/bread exchange, plus 1 fat exchange.)

Biscuit, 2 1/2 in. across	1
Chow mein noodles	1/2 cup
Corn bread, 2 in. cube	1 (2 oz.)
Cracker, round butter type	6
French fried potatoes, 2 in. to 3 1/2 in. long	10 (1 1/2 oz.)
Muffin, plain, small	1
Pancake, 4 in. across	2
Stuffing, bread (prepared)	1/4 cup

2
MEAT LIST

ach serving of meat and substitutes on this list contains about 7 grams of protein. The amount of fat and number of calories varies, depending on what kind of meat or substitute you choose. The list is divided into three parts based on the amount of fat and calories: lean meat, medium-fat meat, and high-fat meat. One ounce (one meat exchange) of each of these includes:

	Carbohydrate (grams)	Protein (grams)	Fat (grams)	Calories
Lean	0	7	3	55
Medium-Fat	0	7	5	75
High-Fat	0	7	8	100

You are encouraged to use more lean and medium-fat meat, poultry, and fish in your meal plan. This will help decrease your fat intake, which may help decrease your risk for heart disease. The items from the high-fat group are high in saturated fat, cholesterol, and calories. You should limit your choices from the high-fat group to three (3) times per week. Meat and substitutes do not contribute any fiber to your meal plan.

🖝 *Meats and meat substitutes that have 400 milligrams or more of sodium per exchange are indicated with this symbol.*

Meats and meat substitutes that have 400 mg or more of sodium if two or more exchanges are eaten are indicated with this symbol.

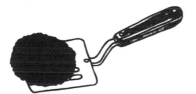

TIPS

1. Bake, roast, broil, grill, or boil these foods rather than frying them with added fat.

2. Use a nonstick pan spray or a nonstick pan to brown or fry these foods.

3. Trim off visible fat before and after cooking.

4. Do not add flour, bread crumbs, coating mixes, or fat to these foods when preparing them.

5. Weigh meat after removing bones and fat, and after cooking. Three ounces of cooked meat is about equal to 4 ounces of raw meat. Some examples of meat portions are:
   2 ounces meat (2 meat exchanges) =
      1 small chicken leg or thigh
      1/2 cup cottage cheese or tuna
   3 ounces meat (3 meat exchanges) =
      1 medium pork chop
      1 small hamburger
      1/2 of a whole chicken breast
      1 unbreaded fish fillet
      cooked meat, about the size of a deck of cards

6. Restaurants usually serve prime cuts of meat, which are high in fat and calories.

LEAN MEAT AND SUBSTITUTES
(One exchange is equal to any one of the following items.)

Beef: USDA Select or Choice grades of lean beef, such as round, sirloin, 1 oz.
and flank steak; tenderloin; and chipped beef 🖋

Pork: Lean pork, such as fresh ham; canned, cured or boiled ham 🖋 1 oz.
Canadian bacon 🖋, tenderloin.

Veal: All cuts are lean except for veal cutlets (ground or cubed). 1 oz.
Examples of lean veal are chops and roasts.

Poultry: Chicken, turkey, Cornish hen (without skin) 1 oz.

Fish: All fresh and frozen fish 1 oz.
Crab, lobster, scallops, shrimp, clams 2 oz.
  (fresh or canned in water)
Oysters 6 medium
Tuna ★ (canned in water) 1/4 cup
Herring ★ (uncreamed or smoked) 1 oz.
Sardines (canned) 2 medium

Wild Game: Venison, rabbit, squirrel 1 oz.
Pheasant, duck, goose (without skin) 1 oz.

Cheese: Any cottage cheese ★ 1/4 cup
Grated parmesan 2 Tbsp.
Diet cheeses 🖋 (with less than 55 calories per ounce) 1 oz.

Other: 95% fat-free luncheon meat 🖋 1 1/2 oz.
Egg whites 3 whites
Egg substitutes with less than 55 calories per 1/2 cup 1/2 cup

---

🖋 *400 mg or more of sodium per exchange*

★ *400 mg or more of sodium if two or more exchanges are eaten*

MEDIUM-FAT MEAT AND SUBSTITUTES
(One exchange is equal to any one of the following items.)

Beef: Most beef products fall into this category. Examples are: all ground 1 oz.
beef, roast (rib, chuck, rump), steak (cubed, Porterhouse, T-bone),
and meatloaf.

Pork: Most pork products fall into this category. Examples are: chops, loin 1 oz.
roast, Boston butt, cutlets.

Lamb: Most lamb products fall into this category. Examples are: chops, 1 oz.
leg, and roast.

Veal: Cutlet (ground or cubed, unbreaded) 1 oz.

Poultry: Chicken (with skin), domestic duck or goose (well drained 1 oz.
of fat), ground turkey

Fish: Tuna ★ (canned in oil and drained) 1/4 cup
Salmon ★ (canned) 1/4 cup

Cheese: Skim or part-skim milk cheeses, such as:
Ricotta 1/4 cup
Mozzarella 1 oz.
Diet cheeses 🖋 (with 56-80 calories per ounce) 1 oz.

Other: 86% fat-free luncheon meat ★ 1 oz.
Egg (high in cholesterol, limit to 3 per week) 1
Egg substitutes with 56-80 calories per 1/4 cup 1/4 cup
Tofu (2 1/2 in. × 2 3/4 in. × 1 in.) 4 oz.
Liver, heart, kidney, sweetbreads 1 oz.
  (high in cholesterol)

🖋 *400 mg or more of sodium per exchange*

400 mg or more of sodium if two or more exchanges are eaten

HIGH-FAT MEAT AND SUBSTITUTES

Remember, these items are high in saturated fat, cholesterol, and calories, and should be used only three (3) times per week.

(One exchange is equal to any one of the following items.)

Beef:	Most USDA Prime cuts of beef, such as ribs, corned beef	1 oz.
Pork:	Spareribs, ground pork, pork sausage 🐾 (patty or link)	1 oz.
Lamb:	Patties (ground lamb)	1 oz.
Fish:	Any fried fish product	1 oz.
Cheese:	All regular cheeses, such as American 🐾, Blue 🐾, Cheddar , Monterey Jack , Swiss	1 oz.
Other:	Luncheon meat 🐾 , such as bologna, salami, pimento loaf	1 oz.
	Sausage 🐾 , such as Polish, Italian smoked	1 oz.
	Knockwurst 🐾	1 oz.
	Bratwurst	1 oz.
	Frankfurter 🐾 (turkey or chicken)	1 frank (10/lb.)
	Peanut butter (contains unsaturated fat)	1 Tbsp.

Count as one high-fat meat plus one fat exchange:

Frankfurter 🐾 (beef, pork, or combination)	1 frank (10/lb.)

🐾 *400 mg or more of sodium per exchange*

400 mg or more of sodium if two or more exchanges are eaten

3
VEGETABLE LIST

Each vegetable serving on this list contains about 5 grams of carbohydrate, 2 grams of protein, and 25 calories. Vegetables contain 2-3 grams of dietary fiber. Vegetables which contain 400 mg or more of sodium per exchange are identified with a 🥓 symbol.

Vegetables are a good source of vitamins and minerals. Fresh and frozen vegetables have more vitamins and less added salt. Rinsing canned vegetables will remove much of the salt.

Unless otherwise noted, the serving size for vegetables (one vegetable exchange) is:

1/2 cup of cooked vegetables or vegetable juice
1 cup of raw vegetables

Artichoke (1/2 medium)
Asparagus
Beans (green, wax, Italian)
Bean sprouts
Beets
Broccoli
Brussels sprouts
Cabbage, cooked
Carrots
Cauliflower
Eggplant
Greens (collard, mustard, turnip)
Kohlrabi
Leeks

Mushrooms, cooked
Okra
Onions
Pea pods
Peppers (green)
Rutabaga
Sauerkraut 🥓
Spinach, cooked
Summer squash (crookneck)
Tomato (one large)
Tomato/vegetable juice 🥓
Turnips
Water chestnuts
Zucchini, cooked

Starchy vegetables such as corn, peas, and potatoes are found on the Starch/Bread List.

🥓 *400 mg or more of sodium per exchange*

4
FRUIT LIST

Each item on this list contains about 15 grams of carbohydrate and 60 calories. Fresh, frozen, and dried fruits have about 2 grams of fiber per exchange. Fruits that have 3 or more grams of fiber per exchange have a ⚘ symbol. Fruit juices contain very little dietary fiber.

The carbohydrate and calorie content for a fruit exchange are based on the usual serving of the most commonly eaten fruits. Use fresh fruits or fruits frozen or canned without sugar added. Whole fruit is more filling than fruit juice and may be a better choice for those who are trying to lose weight. Unless otherwise noted, the serving size for one fruit exchange is:

> 1/2 cup of fresh fruit or fruit juice
> 1/4 cup of dried fruit

FRESH, FROZEN, AND UNSWEETENED CANNED FRUIT

Apple (raw, 2 in. across)	1 apple
Applesauce (unsweetened)	1/2 cup
Apricots (medium, raw)	4 apricots
Apricots (canned)	1/2 cup, or 4 halves
Banana (9 in. long)	1/2 banana
⚘ Blackberries (raw)	3/4 cup
⚘ Blueberries (raw)	3/4 cup
Cantaloupe (5 in. across)	1/3 melon
(cubes)	1 cup
Cherries (large, raw)	12 cherries
Cherries (canned)	1/2 cup
Figs (raw, 2 in. across)	2 figs
Fruit cocktail (canned)	1/2 cup
Grapefruit (medium)	1/2 grapefruit
Grapefruit (segments)	3/4 cup
Grapes (small)	15 grapes
Honeydew melon (medium)	1/8 melon
(cubes)	1 cup
Kiwi (large)	1 kiwi
Mandarin oranges	3/4 cup
Mango (small)	1/2 mango
⚘ Nectarine (2 1/2 in. across)	1 nectarine
Orange (2 1/2 in. across)	1 orange
Papaya	1 cup
Peach (2 3/4 in. across)	1 peach, or 3/4 cup
Peaches (canned)	1/2 cup or 2 halves
Pear	1/2 large, or 1 small
Pears (canned)	1/2 cup, or 2 halves
Persimmon (medium, native)	2 persimmons
Pineapple (raw)	3/4 cup
Pineapple (canned)	1/3 cup
Plum (raw, 2 in. across)	2 plums
⚘ Pomegranate	1/2 pomegranate
⚘ Raspberries (raw)	1 cup
⚘ Strawberries (raw, whole)	1 1/4 cup
⚘ Tangerine (2 1/2 in. across)	2 tangerines
Watermelon (cubes)	1 1/4 cup

DRIED FRUIT

⚘ Apples	4 rings
⚘ Apricots	7 halves
Dates	2 1/2 medium
⚘ Figs	1 1/2
⚘ Prunes	3 medium
Raisins	2 Tbsp.

FRUIT JUICE

Apple juice/cider	1/2 cup
Cranberry juice cocktail	1/3 cup
Grapefruit juice	1/2 cup
Grape juice	1/3 cup
Orange juice	1/2 cup
Pineapple juice	1/2 cup
Prune juice	1/3 cup

⚘ 3 or more grams of fiber per exchange

5
MILK LIST

ach serving of milk or milk products on this list contains about 12 grams of carbohydrate and 8 grams of protein. The amount of fat in milk is measured in percent (%) of butterfat. The calories vary, depending on what kind of milk you choose. The list is divided into three parts based on the amount of fat and calories: skim/very lowfat milk, lowfat milk, and whole milk. One serving (one milk exchange) of each of these includes:

	Carbohydrate (grams)	Protein (grams)	Fat (grams)	Calories
Skim/Very Lowfat	12	8	trace	90
Lowfat	12	8	5	120
Whole	12	8	8	150

Milk is the body's main source of calcium, the mineral needed for growth and repair of bones. Yogurt is also a good source of calcium. Yogurt and many dry or powdered milk products have different amounts of fat. If you have questions about a particular item, read the label to find out the fat and calorie content.

Milk is good to drink, but it can also be added to cereal, and to other foods. Many tasty dishes such as sugar-free pudding are made with milk. Add life to plain yogurt by adding one of your fruit exchanges to it.

SKIM AND VERY LOWFAT MILK

skim milk	1 cup
1/2% milk	1 cup
1% milk	1 cup
lowfat buttermilk	1 cup
evaporated skim milk	1/2 cup
dry nonfat milk	1/3 cup
plain nonfat yogurt	8 oz.

LOWFAT MILK

2% milk	1 cup fluid
plain lowfat yogurt (with added nonfat milk solids)	8 oz.

WHOLE MILK

The whole milk group has much more fat per serving than the skim and lowfat groups. Whole milk has more than 3 1/4% butterfat. Try to limit your choices from the whole milk group as much as possible.

whole milk	1 cup
evaporated whole milk	1/2 cup
whole plain yogurt	8 oz.

6
FAT LIST

Each serving on the fat list contains about 5 grams of fat and 45 calories.

The foods on the fat list contain mostly fat, although some items may also contain a small amount of protein. All fats are high in calories and should be carefully measured. Everyone should modify fat intake by eating unsaturated fats instead of saturated fats. The sodium content of these foods varies widely. Check the label for sodium information.

UNSATURATED FATS

Avocado	1/8 medium
Margarine	1 tsp.
★ Margarine, diet	1 Tbsp.
Mayonnaise	1 tsp.
★ Mayonnaise, reduced-calorie	1 Tbsp.

Nuts and Seeds:

Almonds, dry roasted	6 whole
Cashews, dry roasted	1 Tbsp.
Pecans	2 whole
Peanuts	20 small or 10 large
Walnuts	2 whole
Other nuts	1 Tbsp.
Seeds, pine nuts, sunflower (without shells)	1 Tbsp.
Pumpkin seeds	2 tsp.

Oil (corn, cottonseed, safflower, soybean, sunflower, olive, peanut)	1 tsp.
Olives	10 small or 5 large
Salad dressing, mayonnaise-type	2 tsp.
Salad dressing, mayonnaise-type, reduced-calorie	1 Tbsp.
Salad dressing (oil varieties)	1 Tbsp.

 Salad dressing, reduced-calorie	2 Tbsp.

(Two tablespoons of low-calorie salad dressing is a free food.)

SATURATED FATS

Butter	1 tsp.
★ Bacon	1 slice
Chitterlings	1/2 ounce
Coconut, shredded	2 Tbsp.
Coffee whitener, liquid	2 Tbsp.
Coffee whitener, powder	4 tsp.
Cream (light, coffee, table)	2 Tbsp.
Cream, sour	2 Tbsp.
Cream (heavy, whipping)	1 Tbsp.
Cream cheese	1 Tbsp.
★ Salt pork	1/4 ounce

🖤 400 mg or more of sodium per exchange

★ 400 mg or more of sodium if two or more exchanges are eaten

Index